Wanting to Talk

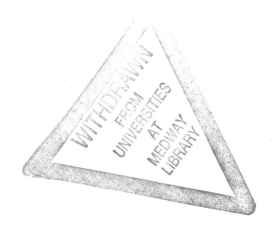

Wanting to Talk

Counselling case studies in communication disorders

Edited by

Diana Syder

Freelance lecturer, therapist and writer

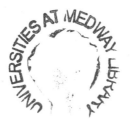

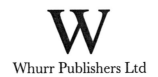

Whurr Publishers Ltd

© 1998 Whurr Publishers Ltd
First published 1998 by
Whurr Publishers Ltd
19b Compton Terrace, London N1 2UN, England

Reprinted 2003 and 2004 (twice)

British Library Cataloguing in Publication Data
A catalogue record for this book is available from the
British Library.

ISBN 1 86156 067 2

Printed and bound in the UK by Athenaeum Press Ltd,
Gateshead, Tyne & Wear

Contents

Contributors

Peter Butcher trained as a clinical psychologist while in Australia. He is currently employed by Tower Hamlets Healthcare NHS Trust as consultant cognitive-behavioural therapist and is also head of Acute Psychology at the Royal London Hospital. In 1985 he co-edited a special issue of the *British Journal of Medical Psychology* entitled 'Sharing Psychological Skills' and he is co-author of *Psychogenic Voice Disorders and Cognitive-Behaviour Therapy* (London: Whurr).

Lesley Cavalli qualified as a speech and language therapist from University College London and has since completed a postgraduate MSc at City University. She is currently working both at the Royal London Hospital as a clinical specialist in voice disorders and at the Department of Clinical Communication Studies, University College London as a lecturer.

Harry Clarke did a one-year counselling foundation course followed by the advanced diploma in counselling and interpersonal skills at the Institute of Education, University of London. He has recently completed the one-year Gestalt counselling skills course at the Gestalt Centre, London. He now works in London as a stroke counsellor at the Clinical Communication Studies Department, City University.

Celia Levy is head of counselling and personal development at the City Literary Institute in London. Initially a speech therapist with an interest in stammering therapy, she now works as a counsellor, trainer and supervisor. Her counselling training began with personal construct psychology but has moved towards a more integrative model, broadly humanistic. Her counselling clients include people with communication disorders.

Peggy Dalton trained as a speech and language therapist and personal construct psychotherapist and counsellor. She has worked as a speech and language therapist, taught and written books on communication disorders and personal construct psychology and now works in independent practice and teaches in London.

Kathryn Lewis is a senior clinical psychologist at the Ryegate Children's Centre (a child development centre) in Sheffield. Her current work involves cognitive and emotional assessment of children with developmental disabilities and neurological problems, individual therapy with children and teenagers, and parent counselling. Her work with children and their families has been strongly influenced by attachment theory and, since she attended courses at the Tavistock Centre in London, psychodynamic theories. She is one of the founders of the Association for Psychotherapies in Learning Disability and is a member of the British Psychological Society.

Allison Pennington is a speech and language therapist with a diploma in clinical hypnosis. She is completing an MMedSci at the University of Sheffield with research into psychogenic voice disorders and hypnosis and also works in adult autism at Thorne House near Doncaster.

Sonia Sharp trained as an educational psychologist at the University of Sheffield after teaching for four years. She worked as principal research fellow on the Sheffield anti-bullying project in the Department of Psychology. She has recently been appointed to the post of chief educational psychologist in Buckinghamshire. She continues to carry out research into bullying and has lectured both nationally and internationally.

Graham Shulman is a child psychotherapist who trained at the Tavistock Clinic, London. He is a member of the autism workshop at the Tavistock Clinic where he has run a group for professionals working in the field of autism, comprising a mixture of therapists from other disciplines. He is also a member of the Tavistock Clinic Infant Observation Research Seminar. He works in the child and family department at Parkside Clinic, an NHS clinic in London.

Diana Syder is a freelance speech and language therapist, lecturer and writer. She worked in the Royal Hallamshire Hospital, Sheffield, for 15 years, initially in neurosurgery and head injury and then in ear, nose and throat, and fluency. For much of that time she was concerned with awareness raising of communication disorders among other hospital staff and also with the personal development of therapists. For seven years she was lecturer and joint head of clinic in the Department of Human Communication Sciences, University of Sheffield.

Preface

'Do not dive into murky waters' said my Microsoft Word 6 handy start-up hint when I first switched on to make a start on this book. Hardly an auspicious beginning! Was someone somewhere trying to tell me something?

It seems that in speech and language therapy we have at last moved beyond debates about whether counselling works and whether it has a place within our work. Instead we have entered the – not so much murky as cloudy – waters of how we might best integrate counselling into our practice and which therapies might be appropriate for which type of client. This book aims to contribute to that process.

The waters of counselling can look decidedly murky if you have dipped your toe in far enough to acquire some information and understanding, but not far enough to know what actually happens in a session or how to apply general principles to an individual client. Confidentiality issues can make this seem an impenetrable area for otherwise curious therapists. Although more therapists are now doing accredited counselling courses and staying on to work within communication disorders and the NHS, some still react to counselling with a mixture of suspicion, awe and fear, often as something that is fine for their clients but not for them, something to feel a little embarrassed about should they find themselves needing the services of a counsellor. I hope that this book will go some way to demystifying the process of counselling (although it is a mysterious process) by giving at least a glimpse of what actually goes on behind those doors once the 'do not disturb' sign goes up and also by revealing something of what is going on in the mind of the counsellor.

In the introduction I address some of the current issues around counselling in speech and language therapy. My original concept was to have a second chapter on the evaluation of counselling interventions but I decided not to have this as a separate section, on the grounds that individual contributors know far more about their assessment materials and principles than I do and that, in any case, assessments make far more sense in the context of particular clients. So each of the case histories describes how a particular model of counselling has been employed with people who have communication problems and each author explains their rationale for assessment and evaluation. The authors were invited to give some background to their own work, to say what has influenced them in their choice of therapy as well as their personal philosophy of therapy. Some authors have chosen to write accounts in the first person, others use the third, the style of reporting being to a large extent part and parcel of the model itself. I have included some authors who do not have a speech and language therapy background in order to compare different approaches.

Any speech and language therapist who becomes a counsellor finds that the specific nature of the disorder becomes less significant. As Celia Levy put it in one of our telephone conversations '. . . you begin to see the person first and foremost as a person, with concerns that are just the same as yours and mine, and who just happens to have a communication disorder.' With this as a working principle there is much less need to classify clients in terms of their disorder, at least for the purposes of counselling. It is the human-ness of each client that counselling addresses. This does not change from a stammerer to a dysphasic, or from you to me. Thus each of the case histories will contain ideas and information that are applicable to your client group, whatever your area or areas of interest. Having said this, I have tried to represent a range of client ages and problems as well as a number of different psychological approaches, simply to interest as wide a group of clinicians as possible.

I use the term 'therapist' to describe a speech and language therapist and 'counsellor' to refer to someone with a counselling or psychotherapy qualification.

Diana Syder
April 1998

Acknowledgements

I would like to thank all the authors who have contributed their time, knowledge and effort to this book. I am amazed that people are willing to fit such extra duties into already hectic schedules and with so little arm-twisting! I would particularly like to thank Celia Levy for agreeing to co-write the chapter on supervision in addition to her case history and for encouraging conversations on the phone.

Without Martin Atkinson, several of these chapters would have remained forever trapped in their floppy discs; his help with transferring data across many different word-processing packages was invaluable. He is also a much better proof-reader than I. I much appreciated Shelagh Brumfitt's helpful comments on the introduction.

Mick Perkins and Sara Howard's *Case Histories in Clinical Linguistics* (Whurr Publishers) gave me the idea in the first place and encouraged me to put a proposal together. Thanks are due to the therapists who have allowed me to use their comments when writing about supervision. On behalf of Harry Clarke I would like to thank Hetty Lynn and Donald Burke. Graham Shulman wishes to thank Maria Rhode for discussions about his chapter.

Chapter 1
Some counselling issues in speech and language therapy

DIANA SYDER

Counselling and psychotherapy – personal and advisory counselling – counselling as part of another role – counselling provision within speech and language therapy – undergraduate and postgraduate training – the place of personal therapy – eclecticism and integration – counselling approaches used in speech and language therapy – counselling approaches not yet widely used in speech and language therapy – assessment, evaluation and documentation of counselling episodes – ethical issues in writing and publishing single case studies.

Counselling and psychotherapy

Sometimes the terms 'counselling' and 'psychotherapy' are used interchangeably. There is no clear-cut distinction between them but there are perceived differences by practitioners, even if there appears to be little agreement on what these are. Some of the suggested distinctions include:

- that psychotherapy aims to produce a change in personality whereas counselling tries to mobilise the resources a person already has for coping with life, without fundamentally changing that person.
- that psychotherapy deals with people who are sufficiently disturbed to warrant treatment within the medical or mental health services whereas counselling tends to deal with people who are functioning more or less normally in society but who want to obtain more out of life and develop personally. Thus counselling takes place in non-medical settings. There is the

special case of health workers in medical settings who practise elements of counselling as part of another role.

- the extent to which the relationship between client and therapist is seen as crucial and a central focus of therapy, or whether the therapist has a more facilitative role in which the client is helped to look at relationships with other people in his or her life. So in psychotherapy, the relationship between the client and the therapist would be an acknowledged part of the experience, with the therapist providing a good, accepting and safe relationship in which the client can explore new ways of being and find a model for future relationships.

The term 'counselling psychologist' refers to a person with a psychology qualification who practises counselling. Both psychotherapy and counselling make use of theoretical models and share similar values and attitudes towards clients.

Personal and advisory counselling

Nichols (1993) describes counselling as having two modes, advisory and personal, and observes that it is common to switch back and forth between the two modes in the course of a session. This certainly applies to much speech and language work, although it might not apply in certain contexts such as a client-centred counselling session. He maintains that the important thing is to be aware of the switch and when it happens because the two require very different styles of interaction. In advisory counselling the main flow of communication is from counsellor to client and in personal counselling it is usually from client to counsellor, although the counsellor will at all times be communicating strong, often non-verbal, messages, to do with acceptance, trust etc. Advisory counselling includes such things as giving information and advice, shaping attitudes and helping behaviour change. Personal counselling explores the experiences, perceptions, feelings and motives of the client and the primary role of the counsellor is to facilitate this in-depth exploration of personal experience.

A lot of what speech and language therapists do falls into the first category. We give information to our clients, we shape healthy attitudes to disease, health and rehabilitation, we model appropriate behaviour and reinforce behaviour change. In that sense we are counselling our clients all the time – it is an activity that flows through everything we do. It is the second category, personal counselling, that has taken so long to be recognised as part of our role.

Counselling as part of another role

Nowadays many professionals use counselling skills as part of a wider role – teachers, doctors, nurses, social workers to name but a few. This can only be desirable. All the communication and interpersonal skills that are useful in the health professions because they enable staff to give psychological support to patients are valuable to human beings generally. Indeed, in America schools that formally teach these basic competencies have shown a drop in truancy, violence and crime and have increased their academic success rates (Goleman 1995).

People have tried to find a label for this level of counselling activity and the term that has become accepted is 'using counselling skills' (Bond 1993). This term is now recognised by the British Association for Counselling and is a useful one for speech and language therapists as well as for students who need reassurance that they are not trespassing on someone else's territory or stepping outside their own role by employing such skills.

Nelson-Jones (1993) distinguishes between a 'counselling relationship', where counselling is the main activity and uses an interview format, and 'helping relationships', which do not necessarily take place in interview settings and where the use of counselling skills is only part of the helper's relationship with the client. Professionals involved in helping relationships carry other primary roles towards their clients and at times may need to act in ways not compatible with the general tenets of a counselling relationship (such as a manager who may need to discipline an employee, a lecturer who may have to assess a student, or a speech and language therapist who may need to teach basic phonetics to a client). It is easy to see that there are occasions when sub-roles can conflict.

In speech and language therapy we 'use counselling skills' but anything beyond this is still, it seems, largely a matter of personal preference and subject to discussion. I would expect energetic debate, even about the nature of our primary role, because we are not a homogeneous group, our primary roles vary both in reality and in our perception of them. Two therapists working in the same clinical area can both see their role very differently, usually related to the relative importance they attach to psychological, cognitive and physical aspects of healthy functioning as well as to the specific skills, knowledge and feelings of confidence they themselves possess. Both therapists are likely to be influenced by how they would like to spend their time with a client as much as by judgements about what would be best for the client.

Speech and language therapists are usually extremely skilled at facilitating and encouraging other people to talk and these skills appear to be well covered within the existing training, but counselling is about more than that. Once you have your client talking and he or she has confided in you, this in itself may be cathartic to some extent but it is unlikely to induce change. Rather it is necessary to do something with the material that is revealed. It is at this stage that speech and language therapists begin to feel out of their depth unless they have received significant further training. Parkinson (1996) puts it this way: that the role of therapist, in addition to having a teaching component, is now seen to require awareness of, and maintenance of, the relationship with a client, which is conducive to positive change. This and all it implies can be seen as the counselling component of the therapist's role. According to Parkinson this requires an ongoing awareness of:

- the client's feelings, thoughts and behaviour;
- the therapist's own thoughts, feelings and behaviour;
- what is happening in the here and now;
- outside events which may be influencing what is currently happening.

Later we will consider whether the above awarenesses are adequately developed in undergraduate training. One confusion that often arises where people have a primary relationship with a client that is not a counselling relationship, and where the counselling relationship is therefore a sub-role, concerns the space, physical and temporal, in which to attend to the psychological elements of care.

The question of formal versus informal settings for counselling has often arisen in conversations with speech and language therapists and, because it implies a basic misunderstanding of the counselling process, I would like to spend some time on it here. Nichols (1993) uses the example of nurses to comment on formal and informal settings for what he calls 'the giving of emotional care'. He cites the case of nurses preferring to talk to patients while they are engaged in some other activity such as helping them to dress or bathing them, on the grounds that the patients '. . . chatter away and tell you their problems'. Nichols makes several succinct points with regard to this approach:

- that if you are simultaneously doing something else, your attention is divided;

- that choosing those situations in itself reflects the nurses' discomfort and anxiety about coping with psychological work as they have built in escape routes;
- that there will be interruptions and distractions;
- that this informal approach downgrades emotional care to something relatively unimportant, something that does not warrant its own space;
- it ignores the client's need for safety, consistency, privacy and confidentiality.

It also ignores the power implications inherent in the situation. The implications of a clothed counsellor talking to a undressed patient hardly bear thinking about. Such occasions, Nichols argues, should be seen as opportunities for complementing structured psychological care. Nurses who counsel clients at bathtime may seem a extreme example but we are all familiar with corresponding scenarios: the chat with the client across his lunch while monitoring a swallowing programme; that throw-away but significant comment from the client on the way to the door and the ensuing conversation with one hand on the door handle; the lengthy diversion in the middle of an assessment; talking to a parent on the way down the corridor or in the waiting room with people pushing past. Such informal settings may be appropriate and desirable occasions for complementing psychological care and again this is something in which speech and language therapists are usually skilled, but how are we to make sure our clients receive more formal, structured psychological care when they need it?

Counselling provision within speech and language therapy

If we do not plan, services are in danger of being patchy across the country and clients may be at the mercy of fate, in the form of the interests and biases of their therapists. This already applies, to some extent, in other areas of our work and we have learned to live with it; we even tell ourselves that such variation is a positive thing and adds to the choices available to clients – which is true in theory though I'm not sure if it is the case in practice. But perhaps when we look at counselling we are dealing with something much more fundamental and something that should not be left to chance, as much for the therapist's benefit as the client's.

When I begin to consider just how we might plan for the formal provision of counselling, questions rather than answers crowd my head. Is counselling of people with communication disorders a specialism within speech and language therapy? Within counselling? Both? Neither? The permutations are extensive. Do we argue that all therapists should be trained counsellors? Is knowledge and understanding of communication disorders unnecessary in order to counsel someone with such a disorder, in which case can we say that the client is better off with a counsellor rather than with a speech and language therapist? Many counsellors would say that people are people and a communication disorder is secondary to those basic human issues that would be the concern of all of us – that people with communication problems are no different in this respect. On the other hand I have also heard speech and language therapists express unease at referring their clients on to counsellors with no speech and language therapy background. They fear the communication disorder will not be taken sufficiently into account, especially where expressive and receptive language problems are present, and that the counsellor will lack strategies for talking, say, to a dysphasic client. Traditionally, people working in fluency and voice have seen counselling as a large part of their primary role, or as being the only means by which to play out the primary role – possibly more so, until recently, than in other adult clinical areas. In paediatrics most counselling has been done with parents rather than children and when children are counselled directly, more often than not this counselling is carried out by a non-speech and language therapist. So the old dilemmas hold as true for counselling training as they do for anything else. Do we restrict precious training resources predominantly to those in fluency and voice? Do we spread resources more thinly and continue to encourage therapists to pay for their own professional development? What is essential and what optional? Certainly the demand for counselling training is there. If nothing else, the shift to community-based care for adults and elderly people in recent years means many more community therapists are questioning what they have to offer to their clients and discovering a need for greater counselling skills and knowledge.

More and more speech and language therapists are qualifying as counsellors. In a survey by Parkinson and Rae (1996) 14% of therapists with five or more years' experience had undertaken formal counsellor qualifications and another 12% were working towards such a qualification. This should make the position easier as long as these counsellors continue to be accessible to clients. Ten years ago it was common to hear stories of therapists having to leave the NHS in order to work in the way they wanted. This was sad but it does seem that there are now more opportunities for therapists to work as counsellors within their mainstream speech and language therapy posts. Some of the responsibility here lies with managers; it is up to them not to drive the counsellors out into private practice.

One possibility would be to follow the model whereby each district employs at least one speech and language therapist who is also a trained counsellor in a specialist counselling post and that all the other therapists are equipped with basic skills. Or speech and language therapy managers could employ trained counsellors with or without speech and language therapy backgrounds to work alongside speech and language therapists. The aim of this would not be to remove responsibility from the rest of us, nor to take away what for some are the prized elements of speech therapists' work. It does have the advantage of creating an obvious referral route and ensuring competence.

It is also desirable that speech and language therapists should be aware of when a client needs more than the 'use of counselling skills' and know where to send the client for that sort of input. This would be another way of doing things, by training therapists to recognise which counselling therapy might help which clients, how to refer them on, and where to refer them. However the last is often a sticking point because resources are not extensive outside the private domain and my impression is that therapists are often not aware of the range and availability of local counselling resources. They do recognise when clients needs further help but often cannot find it for them, or not quickly enough to be useful. They are understandably discouraged from trying again for the next client. To make things worse, people with communication disorders often cannot afford to pay privately for what may be long-term counselling, but neither do they fit many of the services available through the mental health services. Impasse. Meanwhile we still have to deal with the client and his or her distress.

Undergraduate and postgraduate training

Anyone who has written about counselling in speech and language therapy has made a case for a different approach to training and for more of it. Although not wanting to repeat what has already been eloquently said, I do wish to add my voice to those who have already spoken. Davis and Fallowfield (1991) feel that all health care professionals should receive some basic counselling skills training if only to improve communication between staff and patients because the style of interaction used in counselling is beneficial for improved communication, but they expect that counselling in any depth will be carried out by someone who has had appropriate advanced training. Nichols (1993) takes a middle-ground view and says that staff giving psychological care should know what counselling is and be able to offer it at a basic level but should not function as counsellors or therapists. It is as though speech and language therapists sit rather uncomfortably somewhere between needing 'to use counselling skills' and needing to act as counsellors.

Undergraduate training

It could be said speech and language therapists should be given skills up to the level of 'use of counselling skills' as undergraduates, and should be expected to go on from here under their own steam. Surely this is not an option for a discipline in which, even at the point of qualification, therapists are expected to function well beyond this level. For example they are expected to implement behavioural programmes with children and adults, to challenge cognitions, to employ the rudiments of personal construct therapy with fluency clients and to resolve voice disorders of a psychological origin. This suggests they need educating beyond the acquisition of basic communication and interpersonal skills prior to qualifying.

Butcher et al. (1993) support this view, saying '. . . the speech pathologist needs to be more fully trained *in the practical application of psychological approaches* [my italics] in order to work more effectively and efficiently . . .' They are talking about work with psychogenic voice disorders but I would extend their comments to cover all areas of communication disorders. They are arguing that we need to take our basic training beyond the 'use of counselling skills'. They also distinguish between skills that are acquired during the training of speech and language therapists and those that are acquired after qualification. One of the problems is that it is difficult to find a baseline for what is or should be taught as courses vary considerably in both what they teach and how much time is allocated. To complicate things, departments and courses change all the time. Training programmes usually involve the teaching of some interpersonal and basic communication skills and sometimes there is a specific counselling module that serves as an introduction and I doubt any school would claim it to be more than this. Parkinson and Rae (1996) suggest that the issue is no longer how much counselling training should happen at undergraduate level but what sort. I would dearly like to agree with them but feel that, until there are clear guidelines, we should not rest on our laurels.

Butcher et al. unequivocally state that current levels of training at an undergraduate level are insufficient and the training that exists is taught mainly at a theoretical level. They advocate the increased use of illustration with practical applications. I could not agree more and would possibly go further by saying that students should have much more exposure to experiential techniques so that, if nothing else, they get a flavour of what a counselling relationship is like, and more specifically, what it is like to be on the consumer end of a counsellor/client relationship. Parkinson and Rae (1996) make the observation that pre-qualification may not, in fact, be the best time as 'Possibly the student's academic burden does not allow sufficient time or opportunity for self exploration and growth.' Certainly, contemporary academic environments are not conducive to this sort of personal work. They are increasingly competitive places and the distances between students and staff are likely to increase rather than decrease as performance pressures on staff escalate and the number of students continues to increase. Added to this, most training establishments are finding that there is less and less cash available to buy in outside tutors who might be perceived as having no examiner relationship to the student.

When suggestions of increasing the amount of course time spent on practical elements of counselling are put forward at policy meetings in the educational establishments, they are often met with raised eyebrows and other staff waving already crammed course timetables in the air. This is especially so at a time when academic departments are constantly under pressure to reduce their teaching commitment for the sake of research brownie points. Maybe other material would have to be cut, depending on the specific programme and existing provision. If so, why not? Such competences appear to be fundamental. If therapists cannot employ them, they will not be in a position to effectively apply anything else they may have learned in their training. They are also likely to be uncomfortable with circumstances in which they will inevitably find themselves time and time again and this is no stable base from which to operate in a demanding and difficult field. During the Sheffield Supervision Project (see Chapter 10), those therapists who were unhappy to the point of considering leaving the profession (sometimes a hidden issue that brought them into supervision), nearly always lacked the basic strategies and some of the technical skills they needed to handle the counselling elements of their work, although they were experienced and competent therapists. Once given the knowledge and skills, mainly by modelling within the supervision sessions, they became much more settled and confident as well as reporting enjoying their work again.

Postgraduate training

There are many counselling and psychotherapy courses around; they come in all shapes and sizes, from weekends on adult education programmes to both modular and non-modular degree studies. Short courses have been more readily available than longer periods of study, although this has always varied from place to place. We have come a long way in the past 17 years and finding training opportunities has become easier. When I trained, in 1978/9, counselling input to course programmes varied from minimal to non-existent. On my course I don't remember any formal attention being given to communication or interpersonal skills. Learning theory was done in psychology and a smattering of conversational dynamics came from phonetics. That was it. So the only way to develop was to look for whatever post-qualification in-service training courses were on offer. Nowadays there are more flexible course structures on the market to accommodate people who wish to train but who may be working full time and so it is easier for therapists to choose a more cohesive route. In addition the culture has been changing and it is accepted that therapists now take more responsibility for their personal development, including financing it, although there are mixed feelings about this. The question is: how much is personal development a matter of personal choice and how much should be mandatory? How much support for postgraduate education might be expected to come out of training budgets and how much is the therapist expected to pay? Formal psychotherapy and counselling training can cost a formidable amount of money, especially those courses that require the student to undertake both supervision and personal therapy. Even if the therapist can and does pay, it is not always easy to get extended study leave in these days of cutbacks and pruning. We need a clear route, or preferably choice of routes, for therapists considering extending their skills. Not only that, but while working to move things on, we do have to manage with what we've got in the present. I would certainly not want to undermine any therapist's confidence in their level of counselling competence to the extent that they cease to apply the knowledge and skills they have got. Just the opposite, we need to encourage and nurture the existing skills and interest that therapists have in counselling. When the Special Interest Group in Counselling conducted a survey of its membership (Green 1990), the main trends were clearly demonstrated by the 132 responses, of which 75% said client-centred or Rogerian counselling was their predominant influence and 60% personal construct therapy (PCT) whereas the remainder cited a variety of 26 different approaches. Behaviour therapy was mentioned by 23% of therapists but only one mentioned cognitive-behaviour therapy; however, this survey predated Butcher's book (1993) and the figure for cognitive-behaviour therapy might well be higher now.

Surely, as long as the therapist knows enough not to do harm, which of course is easier said than done, it is better for a client to be given some of what he needs, rather than nothing, if that is the option. The danger is that theories and techniques might be applied inadequately and then the approach dismissed as not working. It would also be good to see therapists holding more information about local counselling services inside and outside the NHS which they can pass on to clients and display in waiting areas.

The place of personal therapy

Personal counselling can be seen as part of a wider package of self development, which might include reading, formal courses, short courses and group workshops. Some counselling training courses insist that students enter therapy as part of their preparation to become a counsellor, but not all. Personal counselling often leads people towards wanting to be counsellors themselves and, conversely, it is well known that what often brings people onto counselling courses is their own, sometimes unconscious, need.

It is hard to understand how anyone can be an effective and empathic counsellor, or understand the process, unless he or she has been on the receiving end of a client/counsellor relationship, with all that that implies for the experiencing of power issues, dependency/independency, projections and so on. How can therapists identify their own issues and separate them from a potential client's if they haven't been taught how to, or been challenged about their own behaviour in therapy or in supervision? Personal experience is very valuable. I have often heard hospital workers, after being in hospital themselves, or having a relative hospitalised, say that they come back to work with a fresh eye and a greater feeling for what their patients go through. As a basic principle I make students try on themselves anything they might ask clients to do; to have their case history taken, to complete an S24, a self-characterisation, to keep a voice diary etc. This is not so much to give a partner the opportunity to practise administering such things, but so that the recipient learns what it is like to struggle with questions that may seem irrelevant, or too specific, or not specific enough, to be pinned down for a definite response to something that may be hard to verbalise, to make decisions about what aspects of themselves should be made public and what kept private and so on. My hope is that, having done this, the students are far more likely to acknowledge and deal with these aspects of their clients' behaviour when they arise, not to dismiss them or maybe feel irritated or disappointed when clients arrive with a bare voice diary, two lines of a self-characterisation or a half-completed S24. I believe it also sets up a desirable pattern of extrapolating from personal experience without falling into the trap of assuming that one's own experience is the only experience it is possible to have. Of course we can't experience everything our clients experience. I have never had a fibreoptic tube stuck up my nose, though I've watched plenty of clients go through it. Nor do I want that experience if I can avoid it – it does not look fun. However, I have had other experiences of tubes, needles and anaesthetics as well as complete strangers doing disconcerting things to my body, and I can use those experiences to relate both to people who are afraid of the nasal tube, as well as those who are not.

Surprisingly the literature so far suggests no clear relationship between personal therapy and counsellor efficiency (Dryden et al. 1995) but I would certainly encourage practising speech and language therapists to consider embarking on their own therapy, not only for the benefits it may bring them as individuals, but for what they will learn about being counselled. I learned so much from being in therapy that has since stood me in good stead in my work as a therapist and as a teacher. Of course it is important to recognise that personal therapy on its own does not equip someone to function as a counsellor.

We may be grateful that at long last counselling has moved away from the lunatic fringe of our profession, but it is still regarded with suspicion by some. From time to time I am approached by therapists wanting advice about finding a counsellor and whether or not counselling might help them. A common attitude is that counselling is OK for them (our clients) but not for us (the speech and language therapists). Often there is an element of sheepishness in the therapist's approach, a sense of failure, shame sometimes, self-consciousness certainly. Rarely is it viewed or spoken of as an exciting opportunity, or a sensible form of self-help. How on earth can we recommend something and even practise it with our clients when we feel this way? What does it say about the way we view counselling and the way we view our clients? Parkinson and Rae (1996) suggest that '. . . a possible reluctance to engage in this work may arise from the medical roots of our profession with the emphasis on diagnosis and cure in an expert–client dyad rather than a therapeutic relationship'.

Eclecticism and integration

This is a significant issue for speech and language therapy and it is worth spending some time on it. As we have discussed, many therapists have not undergone formal counselling training but have actively sought out bits and pieces from here, there and everywhere, fitting together whatever was available or necessary over a period of time. They may have done a range of short courses in a number of different therapies, been in therapy themselves, read widely and engaged in other self-development activities. This *ad hoc* approach has been due in part, and probably still is, to training and funding policies in the NHS, which has a tradition of limited funding for postgraduate education and only allowing short periods of study leave. The above description certainly fits me and nowadays I am well aware that my own experience could either be described as wide ranging, or as patchy! This means I must be particularly careful not to overstep what I am equipped to do with clients and with other therapists. Many therapists have been steered into a similar position of eclecticism and we need to work with this rather than condemn it.

'In broad terms, eclectic counsellors borrow the best ideas and techniques from a variety of sources and may do so either systematically or haphazardly, while integrative counsellors try to form a coherent harmonious whole from two or more theories or parts of theories' (Bayne et al. 1994). An integrative approach concentrates on the process of a client and counsellor's work together without relying on any one theory of personality or human development. There is something called an 'integrative process model', which formally attempts to provide a structure for integrating ideas and techniques from a number of sources.

Such an integrative approach is based on the rationale that human beings are too complicated to be explained by any one theory. Some practitioners prefer the term 'integrative' because it suggests a coherence and harmony that is not generally associated with the word 'eclectic' (Hough 1994). It struck me as interesting that, of all the discussions on eclecticism I read in counselling texts while preparing this chapter, none gave much, if any, space to discussing the advantages and disadvantages of the single model approach. This fits with the majority of practical clinical experience in which most practitioners are accustomed to drawing on a range of skills, ideas and models. However, there are some strong arguments against the tendency towards eclecticism in speech and language therapy. Hayhow and Levy (1989) make a persuasive case for avoiding eclecticism in working with stutterers. They believe

> that a theoretical framework should help the therapist understand people in general and themselves and people who stutter in particular, and also provide a model for change. The theory must also help us to understand why speech therapy methods work, so that we are not forced into a position of eclecticism. Many theories that have been used in the past have precisely this shortcoming and so the therapist is forced to abandon her previous convictions or to try to distort the evidence so she can continue with her current practices. Once a comprehensive theory has been found the advantages are apparent: success and failure can be understood within that framework and what was previously inexplicable or put down to client shortcomings can now be understood. For example, within other models the failure to generalise fluency outside the clinic may be attributed to lack of motivation or laziness . . .

While agreeing with the authors that a theoretical understanding is vital and that 'without such a structure, therapy may be reduced to a random series of games and activities' the use of a single model can be restrictive. People do respond differently to different approaches but most communication-disordered clients are not in a position to choose their therapists for their approach. If, say, clients enjoy working with metaphor, or find visualisation powerful, or start talking about their inner child, then it makes sense at least to begin work in that way. Some clients are more engaged by certain activities and interpretations and it makes sense to have the flexibility to go along with whatever works for them. It is not always possible, right at the start of therapy, to predict which model will work best for a particular client, even with sound theoretical understanding.

Hayhow and Levy do recognise that '. . . the ways individual clients respond to the same therapy can be so varied that any poorly conceived theories of stuttering will soon prove inadequate.' In addition, many speech and language therapists work with more than one client group – how are they to choose which single model to train in? We have not yet carried out evaluative or comparative studies on the relative merits of counselling approaches for specific communication disorders and we are not at the stage where we can say, with any authority, which therapies work best for which disorders, although there are some pointers. For example, personal construct therapy and cognitive-behaviour therapy are accepted as being appropriate for fluency work and cognitive-behaviour therapy has been shown to work well with psychogenic voice disorders, but these have not yet been challenged by other therapies. There is a dearth of published cases of the use of hypnosis, gestalt therapy, rational emotive therapy, psychoanalysis, psychodrama, art therapy, music therapy or psychosynthesis with communication disordered clients, to name but a few. We have hardly begun to explore, in a serious way, the potential of non-verbal therapies such as art therapy, although they might be expected to be the most useful to many of our clients. In general there is limited empirical research concerning the use of counselling in speech and language therapy (Parkinson and Rae1996).

So the term 'eclectic therapy' is not necessarily a perjorative one. However, we need to differentiate between an eclecticism that comes from selecting techniques and ideas out of a wide body of coherent knowledge and using those same techniques because they are all we know and because we don't possess a wide bank of knowledge and skills from which to make a choice.

Counselling approaches used in speech and language therapy

Butcher et al. (1993) give an excellent summary of current psychological practice in speech and language therapy. They describe client-centred therapy, personal construct therapy, behaviour therapy and anxiety control training. Those authors who have used these approaches in their case studies for this book show how the basic theoretical principles are applied in practice. When talking about different types of therapy it helps to consider the three main orientations in counselling and psychotherapy. These are:

- psychoanalytical;
- behavioural;
- humanistic.

This can be a simplistic division but it includes the following (Hough 1994):

- psychoanalytical – includes therapies of Freud, Jung, Adler and the object relations theorists.
- behavioural: all therapies linked to learning theories but also nowadays encompassing cognitive therapies such as Ellis's rational emotive therapy.
- humanistic: includes Rogers (person-centred counselling), Perls (Gestalt therapy) and Berne (transactional analysis).

The group that a specific therapy belongs to can sometimes be disputed but these categories do give us a useful structure for considering the dozens of therapies in existence. Many of the psychological approaches shown in the following case histories are familiar to us – at least we know the basic principles, the underlying theories and perhaps some specific techniques – but there are many counselling therapies at the moment not used in speech and language therapy that would seem to be tempting ground for experiment and research. I have always been puzzled by why some counselling approaches have taken off in speech and language therapy while others have not. One theory is that we are happiest with those concrete and relatively directive therapies that most closely approach our own medical model of operation and whose assessment and recording rationale also approximate to our own. This would explain the adoption of PCT and cognitive-behaviour therapy, although not necessarily hypnosis. Hypnosis has now been accepted as one of the psychological approaches to communication disorders, and hypnotic techniques are sometimes used in relaxation work. Training courses are available but it is still relatively rare to come across qualified therapist-hypnotherapists still working within NHS speech and language therapy services.

Counselling approaches not yet widely used in speech and language therapy

It might be useful to summarise the underlying ideas of some counselling approaches that, as yet, do not have a clear role in treating communication disorders and are not otherwise represented in this book. It was difficult to choose which therapies to include and which to leave out – there is a dazzling array available. I have selected those higher profile therapies that I personally know enough about to get a sense of whether or not they might be directly relevant in the treatment of communication disorders. I did try to have Gestalt and art therapy represented but was unsuccessful. There are other omissions. Key word searches of the literature linking individual therapies to communication disorders turn up very little. If there are therapists out there who use specific therapies that have not been included here, I would urge them to start writing up and publishing cases so that, as a profession, we can develop our psychological care of clients.

Gestalt

Gestalt tries to make clients aware of how they block good contacts between their own senses and the environment (Nelson-Jones 1989)

Developed from the work of Fritz Perls it is relatively directive, much more so than, say, client-centred therapy, and focuses on the present rather than the past. It views life as a process whereby, as one gestalt or 'whole' is completed, another begins. So Gestalt therapy introduces the idea of 'closure' or the 'rounding off' of unfinished situations in order to prevent the unfinished business impairing our ability to fully experience anything else (Ernst and Goodison 1988). Gestalt also aims to fill gaps in our awareness by owning projections and the rejected parts of ourselves, thus making ourselves complete people. Gestalt techniques include drama and fantasy work, dream work, empty-chair dialogues and skilful frustration. I am surprised that Gestalt has not made its way into speech and language therapy as it would seem to have many applications. I have successfully used empty-chair experiments and the idea of unfinished business with stammerers and voice clients.

Transactional analysis (TA)

Many therapists will be familiar with the notion of different aspects of our personalities being likened to parent, adult and child ego states. These three ego states are used to explain and predict relationships and behaviour. This approach was originated by Eric Berne (of *Games People Play* fame). TA has four components operating at increasing levels of complexity: structural analysis of ego states, transactional analysis, game analysis and script analysis. It might well be useful for exploring and describing inter- and intra-personal relationships for people with communication disorders as the basic ideas are easy to grasp and use a familiar vocabulary.

Grief therapy

Colin Murray Parkes, in his foreword to Worden (1983), writes that '. . . bereavement is a turning point in personal development, a psycho-social transition that carries an increased risk to physical and mental health. At such times people are more aware than usual of their need for help . . .' and whoever helps them '. . . needs to know the difference between healthy and unhealthy grieving and know how to support the one and avert the other.' This applies not only to bereavement but to loss in all the forms it takes for the people we encounter every working day: loss of health, abilities, skills, hopes, jobs, money, lifestyles, relationships, freedom, self-expression, self-esteem . . . the list goes on. If grief is not dealt with, it is reflected in our mental and physical health; the aphasic client who becomes depressed; the bereaved woman who develops a psychogenic dysphonia; the anger of parents with a severely disabled baby. Grief counselling aims to facilitate uncomplicated grief by supporting the grieving person through the four normal tasks of mourning: to accept the reality of the loss; to experience the pain of grief; to adjust to an environment in which the deceased is missing; to withdraw emotional energy and reinvest it in another relationship (Worden 1983). It is undertaken by trained doctors, nurses, psychologists and social workers. There are also self-help groups of various types where volunteers are supported by professionals or where bereaved people help other bereaved people, either in groups or individual sessions. In this way the grieving person is helped to make a healthy with-drawal from whatever has been lost and to reinvest emotional energy in other relationships and with life in general. There are people for whom grief can be excessive, absent, delayed or prolonged. It can also manifest as a physical symptom. In such instances grief therapy aims to identify and resolve those conflicts that are standing in the way of the completion of mourning.

In speech and language therapy we come across people who are going through the normal stages of grieving as well as those who exhibit signs of pathological grief. Sometimes the process of grieving is directly linked to the presenting condition as in the example of a woman who has a psychogenic dysphonia following the death of her husband. Sometimes we are trying to rehabilitate people who are in the process of grieving their former selves. There would seem to be a great need for grief therapy within speech and language therapy.

Drama therapy and psychodrama

Re-enacting a real or fantasy situation helps explore and resolve current dilemmas. This is usually done as group work in which other people are co-actors. The problem is identified and a specific instance selected by the protagonist and the director. Members of the group are then chosen to act the roles of other people involved in the scene – not only people but animals or inanimate objects as well. In this way the protagonist can express feelings directly, rather than simply talking about them. Pioneered by JL Moreno, it uses sculpt-ing, role reversal, empty chair, soliloquy, doubling and the acting out of dreams. I do not know of any qualified drama therapists working in speech and language therapy, which does not mean there are none, but they must be thin on the ground. I find some of the tech-niques very useful and powerful. I do use the empty chair technique. For example, a 29-year-old stammerer came into his session overtly agitated and began to talk about the angry feelings he had towards his teacher, who had humiliated him in class when he was a small boy. By acting the part of himself as a small boy, and that of his teacher, he was able to let out some of those angry feelings and in the process of doing this he also discovered both hurt and puzzled feelings towards her. He was able to say important things to 'her' before we finished the exercise. Immediately afterwards he reported feeling 'great', 'calmer', with increased self-confidence and self-respect. Empty chair dialogues can also be useful when a client is saying something like 'A bit of me thinks x, but another bit of me thinks y.' In this instance clients can have a dialogue between the two aspects of themselves that are represented. It is a good way to help clients clarify their thoughts and feelings and to make important decisions.

Family therapy

Most paediatric therapists know something about family therapy but it can be useful for adults too. Therapy takes place with all members of the family present and relationship problems are seen not as the fault of one individual but as the result of the system that operates within the family, for which all members share responsibility. All are seen as playing their part in setting up and maintaining the problem, often loading it onto an individual, the scapegoat. It is used for helping dysfunctional families recognise what motivates their behaviour and what strategies they use to maintain it. Family therapy is usually available in children's mental health services. It is easy to recognise a role for family therapy with children who have communication disorders with or without compounding problems, but it might also have a place where one member of a family has a head injury or other acquired communication problem.

Co-counselling

This was very popular in my region (Sheffield) in the 1980s among speech and language therapists. Two people agree to work together, with one being the counsellor and the other the client, for an agreed period of time, usually anything from 15 to 30 minutes or longer. At the end of this time they switch roles and continue for an equal amount of time. They will use basic listening skills and response modes and offer focused attention, and some strategies for intensifying feelings. It is an accessible form of therapy and because there is a mutual contract and disclosure, both parties operate as equals. The disadvantages are that it can be superficial and therefore not suitable for deep-seated concerns and explorations. It does not have a place for confrontation and it can be difficult for participants to swap roles, especially when the client is engrossed in demanding material. It may conceivably have a role in speech and language therapy as a form of mutual support or peer supervision between therapists.

Art therapy

Art therapy uses visual media in a therapeutic setting. Artists and therapists continually debate the boundaries between art and therapy. Most art therapists are people who have done an arts degree followed by a – usually shorter – training period in art therapy (for example, one year). There are good arguments for reversing that balance and saying that practitioners should have a sounder therapeutic background and a shorter arts course, because they are acting primarily as therapists, not artists. Similar arguments exist in the even newer concept of writing therapy where creative writing, both poetry and prose, is used in a therapeutic context. Art therapy as a discrete entity has only been in this country since the 1940s and it was not until the 1980s that the first courses appeared. Like all young disciplines it faces the task of defining and refining itself.

The division between what is art and what is therapy depends on whether the process or some final product is seen as paramount. Most, if not all, creative writing is therapeutic but not all writing is art. Of course 'art' (not to mention 'Art') is a slippery concept in the first place. Dalley (1989) says of art therapy

> . . . art activity undertaken in a therapy setting with clear corrective or treatment aims, in the presence of a therapist, has a different purpose and objective. In therapy, the person and process become more important, as art is used as a means of non-verbal communication. Put more elaborately, art activity provides a concrete rather than verbal medium through which a person can achieve both conscious and unconscious expression, and can be used as a valuable agent for therapeutic change.

This is significantly different from artistic activities used as a distraction from inner problems, which though they are valuable for that, are likely to have short term benefits only. Having said that we should not underestimate the deep therapeutic effect of having a channel for expressing ourselves. We are sadly only too familiar with what can happen to people who do not have a means of doing that.

In an art therapy session the client is encouraged to make the art work and will spend some time on this. Fundamental thoughts and feelings, even ones the client cannot verbalise (and may not even be conscious of), can find expression in visual images. The therapist will then focus the client on elements of the picture such as images, colours, spacing and relative size of objects. This provokes awareness and the client is then helped to relate those elements and aware-nesses to his or her current life situation: the client is able to find a meaning for the picture in terms of his or her own life. For non-verbal clients especially there is still the predicament of the verbal medium used in the second phase of an art therapy session, but we might hope that this is made a little easier because at least some abstractions have been made concrete in the form of the picture, and are therefore easier for, say, a dysphasic person to deal with.

Art therapy has been widely used with children but there are few posts in the NHS or education in the UK and many therapists work privately. They tend to work in mental health settings, with psychogeriatric patients, severe physical handicap, learning disabili-ties and with people in prison. Some use group work.

It is astonishing that we do not have more bridges between art therapy and our own discipline when there is so much ground on which to work. We cling to verbal techniques, whatever we say to the contrary, and then express surprise when our clients do the same! But then we live in a society where verbal facility, particularly spoken, is prized above all else. We know this only too well: we spend hours and hours teaching clients and students about how many other processes are involved in communicating, besides speech. None the less our own training does encourage us to concentrate on words. Having done what must be hundreds of interviews for student places I am aware that to a significant extent, we select for verbal abilities. It would be good to see more non-verbal techniques taught to undergraduates, or even postgraduates.

Psychoanalysis and psychodynamic counselling

This is an important psychological approach and although both Kathryn Lewis and Graham Shulman expand on the basic ideas in their chapters this summary may be useful for therapists who are unfamiliar with the fundamental ideas. In general, psychoanalysis refers to long-term, intensive (daily or several times a week) sessions, whereas psychodynamic counselling is shorter and less intensive but uses the same theoretical base. Both reflect a theoretical model of personality that has its roots in the work of Freud and has influenced much twentieth-century thought. 'Psychodynamic refers to the way in which the psyche (as mind/emotions/spirit/self) is seen as active and not static' (Jacobs 1989). It takes account of the relationships we carry within ourselves, between aspects of ourselves. '. . . we can just as easily love, hate or fear parts of ourselves as we can other people' (Jacobs 1989). Different authorities have used different terms to talk about these relationships, such as Freud's 'id', 'ego' and 'super ego'; Jung's 'shadow', 'animus' and 'anima' and Winnicott's 'true' and 'false' selves. These internal facets are sometimes called 'objects' and Freudian theory has the alternative name of object-relations theory in some of the literature.

Objects can also be parts of the body as well as non-human, for example, toys. Internal objects may also be formed by the way a child sees others, not only by relationships to external things, so a psychodynamic approach views fantasies as a valid part of the child's reality and the psyche as a result of the interplay between parents as they actually are or were and the parents as they are/were experienced by the child, especially at times of stress.

So psychodynamic therapy takes account of the interrelationship of internal and external worlds, regression under stress, object relations, the unconscious, the significance of the past and its repetition in the present, the transference relationship (both positive and negative) between client and counsellor, the value of failure on the part of the therapist (the unavoidable failure by the therapist to provide the 'perfect relationship' for the client but in a setting where it can be brought out into the open), the use of endings, the importance of understanding resistance and the rule of abstinence (the deliberate holding back by the therapist in order to encourage the client to speak and explore more) (Jacobs 1989). Transference and counter-transference is probably dealt with more overtly in this therapy than other approaches and when resistance is encountered it is seen as important to understand the origins and reasons for the resistance.

Assessment, evaluation and documentation of counselling episodes

If we are to present and publish more of our counselling experiences with clients, then we need the tools for recording, analysing and evaluating those experiences. Counselling, like speech and language therapy, is a complex process and answering the question 'does it work?' is not as easy or straightforward as we might wish it to be, or as it might appear to other disciplines. This is as true for a single client's progress as it is for the evaluation of interventions with types of disorders. We know this with regard to many other therapeutic interventions. It remains a challenge to devise measures that are sensitive and effective enough to pick out what are sometimes subtle changes in clients. In all areas of speech and language therapy, this has been a long and laborious process and in the past 20 years there has been a proliferation of tests and assessments of all types, each having its own strengths and weaknesses. There is no definitive assessment, so that whatever your speciality, you must choose a test according to your philosophy of therapy and the task in hand. In the same way, different psychological approaches have their own philosophies of assessment and their own preferred measurement tools. It's easy enough to get an idea of the range and number of these by skimming through the test catalogues.

In trying to find measures for the counselling elements of our work we are bound to encounter all the difficulties met by counsellors working in other fields and clinical wisdom would tell us to expect some additional ones, for example as a consequence of working with language impaired clients. In counselling research it is acknowledged that there are some methodological difficulties that make it hard to evaluate outcomes (McLeod 1994). Again, they are not dissimilar to problems already encountered in evaluating various speech and language therapies. For example one of the most serious difficulties for people carrying out research is how to rule out the effects of spontaneous recovery. Although single case-study methodology has also now evolved its own ways of dealing with the problem of spontaneous recovery, most of the histories in this book were not specifically undertaken as research studies. Rather, contributors were asked to describe and demonstrate the process of their work in whatever way they chose to do so, but they were asked to talk, where possible, about their chosen recording and evaluation methods. The basic options are summarised below (from McLeod 1994).

Standardised inventories

These usually invite the client to respond to batteries of questions and ratings. You may have heard of or be familiar with some of them, such as the Minnesota Multiphasic Personality Inventory (MMPI), the Beck Depression Inventory (BDI) and the Hopkins Symptom Checklist. Others include the Rosenberg Test of Self Esteem (Rosenberg 1965) and the State-Trait Anxiety Questionnaire. They give before and after measures and can be used at follow-up. Butcher et al. (1993) draw our attention to the following four useful questionnaires: Snaith's (1981) Irritability-Anxiety Depression Scale as a screening device; the Beck Depression Inventory (Beck et al.1987) for assessing the degree of depression; the

Assertiveness Schedule developed by Rathus (1973) to assess levels of social confidence and assertiveness; and the Dysfunctional Attitude Scale (DAS), which measures psychological strengths and areas of emotional vulnerability, such as approval, love, achievement, perfectionism, entitlement, omnipotence and autonomy, and helps to identify the contribution of wrong thinking to an individual's problems. A self-scoring DAS is published by Burns (1980). They are all verbal tests. I was recently involved in preparing material for the VASES (Visual Analog Self Esteem Scale), a non-verbal picture test of self-esteem (Brumfitt and Sheeran 1998), which is likely to be useful with many of our our not-so-verbal clients.

Client satisfaction questionnaires

These are usually administered at the end of therapy or at follow-up and enable the counsellor to get an overall impression of how the client felt about the counselling, but they are less useful for teasing out specific dynamics within that process. It is interesting that, as speech and language therapists, we frequently ask clients to fill in this sort of information after intensive groups, say, but would be unlikely to request the same after a standard block of therapy.

Ratings of target symptoms

These can be made either by a client or a clinician. They appraise the change in terms of the alterations in concrete and specific problems that brought the client into therapy in the first place. This is sometimes called 'goal attainment scaling'. Again this is something with which we are familiar and regularly use both formally and informally. Such assessments can be difficult when the issues that are initially important to the client change as a result of the therapy and as the client gains more insight into their situation and themselves. Achieving fluency may be overridingly important to a stammerer who is new to therapy but may become less so as time goes on, being superseded by issues such as 'getting on with my life', 'having a better quality of relationships' and 'being confident'. Two formal tests of this type are the Battle Target Complaints (Battle et al. 1966) and the Personal Questionnaire (Shapiro 1961).

Behavioural methods

These can be sensitive and would include diary keeping, recording things like number of situations avoided and fluency counts for stammerers, number of cigarettes smoked, trips out of the home.

Structured interviews by expert clinicians

These usually take at least an hour of the clinician's and the client's time as well as careful training of inteviewers. Examples are the Psychiatric States Schedule, PSS (Spitzer et al. 1970) and the Structured and Scaled Interview to Assess Maladjustment, SSIAM (Gurland 1972).

Ratings by significant others

Close carers or colleagues rate the client's behaviours. This can provide a detailed picture of behaviour, thoughts and feelings. It does depend on how much information the person has about the client and it can be difficult to get at subtle changes or internal factors. This type of evaluation is already widely used within speech and language therapy, particularly where the clients are severely verbally impaired or where the client is a young child.

Ratings by therapists

This can be done in parallel with independent ratings by an expert assessor or with those of the client. Where client and counsellor ratings have been compared it would appear that counsellors are more cautious in their evaluations of change than the clients are (McLeod 1994).

Cost/benefit analyses and cost effectiveness studies

Some third party provides the criteria used for evaluation – usually the body paying for the therapy. Such criteria might include things like the number of days' sick leave in a staff counselling scheme, reduction of student dropout rate following the start of a student counselling service, reduction of number of visits to a GP after seeing a practice counsellor. Cost effectiveness would consider relative cost merits of different types of intervention such as long-term versus short-term therapy. This type of analysis is likely to sit uncomfortably alongside the client-centred basis at the core of a counsellor's work. Following increased demands from management that they increase the number of clients seen, therapists are therefore forced to reduce the number of sessions available to any one client and this can lead therapists to feel they are having to compromise both their personal and professional standards. What is best for the client is no longer the main criteria for evaluation of intervention.

In counselling as in speech and language therapy, there are myriad assessment tools available and it can be daunting to select those that will be the most appropriate for a particular piece of work as well as to justify that selection to other people. In both disciplines there is still a tendency for teams of clinicians and researchers to develop their own local tools, tailor-making them for the job in hand. This must result in much reinventing and makes the issue even more confusing for less experienced researchers and documentors.

For as long as we have sought to satisfy the rigorous demands of the scientific and medical communities, we have refined our measurement tools and have sensibly directed our attention to those parameters that more easily lend themselves to investigation. We choose criteria for evaluation that will satisfy the publishers of journals – we have to: anything else would never see the light of day, no matter how practically useful it might be. Much of what is therapeutically valuable, however, happens at levels that are so subtle they are intrinsically bound up with things that are hard to measure, such as the quality of the relationship between client and therapist. At the most practical level, a client is less likely to return for a second, third or fourth appointment if he doesn't like you, although the dynamics that determine this are hard to identify and almost impossible to quantify. Whereas speech and language therapists are familiar with endless cognitive and linguistic tests, we are less comfortable with, and have usually had less practice at, assessing thinking, feeling and subjective experience. We need to begin to accord these criteria some respectability and resist the temptation to dismiss them as irrelevant or as being side issues incidental to our main therapeutic activity. We must find a way of talking about these parameters and allow them into our accounts to each other of our clinical experiences. This will not be easy; as a group we have spent a long time aiming for detachment and objectivity, doing our best to subtract the personal from our clinical practice and then trying to analyse what is left. It does not take long to teach someone do this. At the beginning of their academic courses, first year student essays contain many personal opinions and statements. By the end of that first year such statements are few and far between as students learn to use the third person, to quote authors and never to use the dreaded 'I'. Final year clinical students easily get confused when asked to integrate objective knowledge with 'I' experience and knowledge. It can be a real uphill struggle to get them to trust and value this sort of knowing. Sometimes students misinterpret our demands that they develop professionalism as meaning that they are expected to put their real selves into some sort of suspended animation and that when they come into the clinic they must deny or hide their true thoughts and feelings for the greater good of the client. In a sense they are expected to do this – they have to learn to separate their own thoughts and feelings from the client's – but these same thoughts and feelings are a measure and indicator of what is going on in the partnership between themselves and the client. In speech and language therapy we have denied ourselves legal access to this valuable information whereas subjective and qualitative tools do have their place in the counselling community and are accepted as valid ways of describing processes, both clinically and in research. The more we counsel our clients, the more we need ways of recording all aspects of what is going on and the more we need to bring personal accounts alongside those forms of information with which we are more familiar and more comfortable.

We can learn a lot from counselling research that has focused on the process of therapy and struggled with the difficult task of producing tools that enable process to be recorded and analysed. It is sometimes helpful to view the analysis of process as discovering the route by which a client moves from point A to point B, as opposed to simply identifying and measuring the start and end points themselves although, of course, even measuring end points is no easy task. Traditionally speech and language therapy has been more concerned with start and end points and we have much to learn about the mapping and measurement of processes that occur in between. These phenomena are difficult to measure because some of them occur inside the client's head, some in the therapist's head and some are the result of the chemistry between the two. They are elusive and not easy to pin down, nor is it easy to keep track of them. Not only that, but the very attempt to do so tends to interrupt, impede or alter the very processes we are wishing to study. It may help to think of this as investigating what is happening inside the therapy, not only what each of the participants is doing, but also what each is thinking, feeling and experiencing. McLeod (1994) calls this 'the interior of therapy'. The following are ways of accessing the interior:

- *Client accounts* ask the client to keep a record of their therapy experiences, often in the form of a diary. We are familiar with diary keeping in speech and language therapy but it is usually used as a diagnostic tool, or for giving clients insight into their own patterns of symptomatic behaviour.
- *In-depth interviews* of clients by researchers have also been used, sometimes across a total period of therapy, sometimes focusing on particular sessions or episodes, for example 'feeling understood' (Bachelor 1988), things they found helpful or hindering

(Berzon et al. 1963), or the most important events in therapy (Bloch et al. 1979) and all three techniques are cited in McLeod (1994). Data obtained in this way can be difficult to organise, collate and interpret, especially for inexperienced practitioners. It can be hard to identify key events or themes, especially across a long period of time. To complicate things, clients and therapists are likely to edit and select from their experience, no matter how hard they try not to do this.

- *Observations of audio or video recording* have offered opportunities to get inside the therapy. This method can give standardised quantitative data and reveal sequences of behaviour. However, the researcher does not gain access to the internal processes of either party.

- There are a number of *questionnaires and rating scales* that can be completed by the client and/or therapist, usually at the end of sessions, looking at aspects of therapy such as warmth and genuineness, depth of experiencing, vocal patterns, perceptual processing, verbal behaviour, client exploration, therapist exploration, psychic distress, client participation, hostility or dependency, therapist warmth and others. However, they are designed for use over a whole session or several sessions and are of little use when wishing to study parts of sessions or specific events and behaviours within sessions. Examples are the Working Alliance Inventory (WAI) (Horvath and Greenberg, 1996, 1989); the Barrett–Lennard Relationship Inventory (BLRI), which looks at level of regard, congruence, empathic understanding and unconditionality of regard; the Therapy Session Report (Orlinsky and Howard 1975, 1986) dealing with affective quality of session, goal attainment and relatedness; the Session Evaluation Questionnaire (SEQ) (Stiles 1980; Stiles and Snow 1984) looks at depth, smoothness, positivity and arousal (all in McLeod 1994).

- *Interpersonal process recall* (IPR) is a powerful tool for gaining access to the inner worlds of both client and counsellor, or indeed of any two people who happen to be interacting. It is not to be confused with the identical acronym for independent performance review. Interpersonal process recall was developed in the 1960s by Norman Kagan, an American professor of education. Video or audiotapes of sessions are reviewed by the counsellor (recaller) and supervisor (enquirer). The recaller is encouraged by the enquirer's open question techniques to remember and analyse aspects of the interaction that he may not have had time for in the original session. The method has since been applied to counsellor training, supervision, therapy and research (Kagan 1994) and is described more fully in Chapter 10.

- *Self-monitoring* has also been used. Barkham and Shapiro (1986) asked clients to press a concealed button whenever they felt they were being understood during an episode of therapy. This does run the risk of interfering with the process of therapy by asking the client to step back and comment on his own process at the same time as getting on with it. For a while now, speech and language therapists, particularly those involved in training, have puzzled over the tangled question of what exactly it is that a good therapist does that a well-intentioned lay person does not. We have tried to identify the hundred small strategies that therapists use when speaking to their clients. In recent times it has become important to have answers to this question in response to the idea of volunteers, assistants and helpers. Being able to describe such behaviours would also help enormously in monitoring the development of students and designing training courses. Elliott (1987) (cited in McLeod 1994) identified more than 20 different systems used in the literature for classifying counsellor response modes. Those that appear most are: questioning, advising, giving information, minimal responding, reflecting, interpretation, self-disclosure, reassessing, confrontation and acknowledgment. In an attempt to assess the intention of the therapist in choosing a response, rather than the presence or absence of a certain response, Hill and O'Grady (1985) listed 19 therapist intentions: to set limits, get information, give information, support, focus, clarify, convey hope, cathart, identify maladaptive cognitions, give feedback on insight, promote change, reinforce change, overcome resistance, challenge, resolve problems in the therapeutic relationship and deal with therapist needs.

Although I have not yet had an opportunity to try it, I am drawn to Yalom's idea of inviting clients for a year follow-up session during which he plays the client a tape recording of their first session and listens for the clients' reactions to their former selves, to the 'different person' they then were. Often the changes are so subtle they would be unlikely to show up on outcome measures, yet they indicate significant changes in personhood (Yalom 1989).

From the above we can see that the task of recording and analysing exists at several levels, depending on the rationale and unit of analysis, whether it be the whole of a period of therapy, single sessions, significant sections or micro-segments (therapist and client utterances within sessions), and different tools have been evolved to cater for the different levels. In the case histories that follow we shall see how these methods, or combinations of methods, have been used with clients.

Ethical issues in writing and publishing single case studies

When writing up and publishing a counselling case history there are ethical issues to be considered, many of which involve confidentiality. Consent should be obtained from the client to use the material from sessions, whether it is case history information or transcripts/parts of transcripts. Any biographical information that might compromise the client's anonymity should either be omitted altogether or disguised. For example a client's profession might be amended to a different but similar one and, of course, names must be changed. This sounds easy but in practice it can be very difficult to disguise someone's true identity. It is surprising how little information we need in order to recognise someone we know. Written material and data referring to the client, whether it be on disc, tape or paper, should also be protected with the source of biographical information limited to as few copies as possible and kept in a safe place, just as would normally be the case with a client's notes in any clinical setting. It is normal to explain to clients the strategies that will be employed to protect their confidentiality. One strategy is to let clients see the scripts before publication so they can check it for identity clues, but this may alter some of the dynamics between client and counsellor and if the therapy has already finished there is little chance to work the issues through. Some clients are pleased to be approached with this sort of request they feel special, or they want to help or in some way express gratitude for help they've received. All of this may affect the therapy itself and may be need to be addressed within the therapy.

It can be harder for the therapist to make an unbiased relationship with the client if she knows she is documenting him in this way. In a sense the client is special to her, but for reasons not solely concerned with the well being of the client. It may be hard not to consciously or unconsciously manipulate the therapy in some way, either to make it fit certain theories, or to make it fit into a certain time span, say to fit service policies or publication deadlines. There can be conflicting interests when the therapist has obligations to the client, who needs work to proceed at a pace that meets his needs, and also to policies of service provision that may need the work to be completed within a certain timescale.

It makes sense – and is in any case good practice – to ask clients' permission to use their stories for research material or publication as soon as possible and preferably right at the start of the study. If you have already invested a lot of thought and care into documenting a case up to publication standard it can be very difficult and frustrating if the client declines to be involved and it can invoke a conflict between differing roles for the therapist.

The process of documentation itself may intrude on the therapy in some way. Taping sessions is often done for supervision purposes and clients do not usually have a problem with this. If you are asking the client to document the process, however, or if you wish to re-administer tests at certain intervals, this might well interfere with the flow of therapy. It may induce anxieties and expectations on behalf of the client as to whether they have made enough progress. Also asking a client to step back and verbalise about the process of therapy at particular points, be they regular time intervals or related to what is happening in the therapy, may make them feel they have to make sense of what is going on for them at any one point, which may not be possible or desirable. The intentions of this sort of accounting need to be carefully explained to the client but it is hard to rule out their effect.

When the researcher is a third party and not the therapist then a whole new set of dynamics and issues are introduced for all concerned and may give rise to a conflict of interests. Happily this was not an issue for the studies in this book as all the people documenting the cases were therapists to the clients in question. Most institutions have their own ethical committees to vet research proposals and maintain standards of practice. The Royal College of Speech and Language Therapists (RCSLT) and British Psychological Society (BPS) also publish their professional ethical guidelines. For the sort of single case studies in this book it is unlikely to be necessary to consult such committees. For those wishing to read further on ethical issues in counselling research, McLeod (1994) gives a comprehensive practical account, both for single case design and other methodologies.

Chapter 2
Mark: relationship problems for a 13 year old with severe hearing impairment

PEGGY DALTON

Introduction – integrating counselling and speech and language therapy – a personal construct approach to counselling – special issues for hearing-impaired adolescents – issues of confidentiality – the client's story – exploring Mark's view of himself and his world – the process of counselling Mark over a six-month period – preparing for the future – reflections – one young person's experience of hearing loss.

Introduction

I was taken to task by a speech and language therapy colleague some time after the publication of *Counselling People with Communication Problems* (Dalton 1994). She wanted to know why I had not included work with people with hearing impairment in the book. I feebly directed her to the preface, where I stated that hearing impairment, learning difficulties and autism seemed areas of such range and complexity that they warranted a separate volume for each and that they deserved a specialist author with rich experience in these fields that I did not possess. I am not at all sure that she was satisfied with my response and the question stayed with me. I am pleased to have the opportunity to try to make up for my omission.

Integrating counselling and speech and language therapy

Like many of my colleagues who had no element of counselling in their training, I found myself feeling inadequate to deal with the many psychological problems that can arise alongside difficulties with speech, voice, fluency and the trauma that often accompanies neuro-logical impairment. I began looking for a framework within which I could learn more a few years after I qualified. I was attracted to client-centred and cognitive-behavioural therapy in particular but it was reading Fay Fransella's *Personal Change and Reconstruction* (1972) that inspired me to study personal construct psychology more deeply.

I was working mainly with people who stuttered at the time. The idea of approaching the clients' difficulties with the change from dysfluency to fluency and continuing that change over time in terms of the problem of establishing a new role, rather than simply a new pattern of speech, made great sense. As I grew more familiar with the theory its application to work with all clients became clear. The philosophy behind Kelly's work, with its emphasis on our capacity to move on from the constraints of our biographies, seemed to me to offer more to those in trouble than any other approach I had encountered.

I undertook the equivalent of what is now the foundation course in personal construct psychology (PCP) and it was our group who asked for more and around whom Fay Fransella developed the first advanced course. In the meantime the Centre for Personal Construct Psychology was created and within a few years the Diploma in PCP (psychotherapy and counselling) became estab-lished. I have been involved in training courses ever since where there is always a healthy contingent of speech and language thera-pists among the participants.

A personal construct approach to counselling

At the heart of personal construct counselling, as of most approaches, lies respect for the clients' own views of themselves, their worlds and their problems. However baffling, even detrimental to themselves those views may appear to be on first encountering them, the coun-sellor will accept them as valid, for the time at least. They represent theories that have evolved through personal experience and are at present the best way they know of making sense of their lives. Until we understand something of that experience we cannot know how the person has come to construe things as he or she does, and we must not assume that we can readily provide more effective alternatives.

Kelly's approach to counselling and psychotherapy, as described in *The Psychology of Personal Constructs* (1955/1991)), is based on his understanding of people as continually striving to make sense of their worlds and their place in them, in order to anticipate events and know how to deal with them. To begin with, our limited experience means that there are few alternatives open to us and we are dependent on others to fulfil our basic needs for food, warmth and comfort. As our experience increases we are able to make more choices and experiment with our environment. Kelly speaks of us as 'scientists', testing out our theories. We have only to observe very young children to recognise that much of their activity is concerned with just such experimentation: manipulating objects to roll or make a noise, crying to summon attention, exploring their toes to discover what they can do with them.

If all goes well young people will continue to experiment in more adventurous ways and build on experience so that their anticipations serve them well and they are able to be flexible when new 'evidence' comes their way. There are limitations for all of us from the limitations of our environments. A person brought up in straitened circumstances will not have the same sort of choices to make as one with the opportunity for richer experience. It may be, however, that the former develops greater ingenuity in fending for himself or herself while the latter is 'spoilt for choice'. Being brought up as an only child is clearly different from growing up in a large family. However, each singleton or member of a large family will make something individual of his or her experience.

The important thing from a PCP point of view is that the way in which we construe events is not carved in stone. All of us are capable of change, of reconstruction. Often, when adults choose to undergo counselling they are aware that they are 'stuck'. Their theories really are not serving them well and they are continually failing to predict what others, even they themselves, will do. Having said that we can all change, however, that does not mean that the task will be easy. Some changes, particularly those related to long and deeply held beliefs and feelings, will be very threatening.

Apparently simple changes in behaviour, such as speaking fluently instead of stuttering, producing the voice in a different way, are very often linked with considerable changes in self-perception and so are more radical than they seem.

Children, on the whole, are referred by others for counselling. Parents, teachers and others find their behaviour or their attitudes troubling. The young people challenge the adults' notions of how a child should be or cast into doubt their own effectiveness as carers. While some children may have a feeling of being in the wrong, others may make no sense of the complaints about them and have no wish for change in themselves.

It is essential, therefore, that before we attempt to encourage change in our clients we make a careful exploration of how they experience their worlds, how they make sense of themselves and others and the very personal meaning to them of the difficulties they present. PCP is especially rich in procedures for such exploration and we shall return to these. First, however, we need to look at aspects of the theory that will clarify what is meant by 'construing', how we develop a system of constructs and some of the processes involved in the development of our experiencing. (For fuller expositions of Kelly's theory see Fransella and Dalton 1990; Dalton and Dunnett 1992.)

The construing system

Kelly describes how we try to make sense of things by a process of comparison and contrast. We construe one person perhaps as like someone familiar to us in being 'easygoing', while a second is 'uptight'. One situation we have experienced has been 'comfortable', another 'anxiety-making' and we may anticipate that a third, new situation will be like the second because it is in a strange place and the people involved are unfriendly. Such bipolar discriminations are constructs. It should be stressed that constructs are not simply verbalised thoughts. We construe through visual perception (light versus dark), hearing (harsh versus mellow), touch (soft versus hard) and smell (sweet versus acrid). Our behaviour itself is seen as an aspect of construing in that by 'behaving' we seek to test out our expectations of the outcome of an action. Many of our constructs are at a low level of awareness and may only be evoked in the form of a gut reaction of fear or pleasure, for example, when we meet someone for the first time who reminds us of an earlier encounter.

Such constructs are seen as linked together to form networks, as where the person we construe as 'easygoing' rather than 'uptight' may also seem 'friendly' rather than 'cold', 'approachable' rather than 'offputting' and so on. Some constructs will be at a higher level of meaning than others. 'Isolated' versus 'feeling of belonging', for instance, clearly has a wealth of possible meanings, whereas 'lives alone' (versus 'lives with others') may be seen as just one aspect of isolation and is therefore said to be subordinate to isolated/belonging. Constructs that are of great significance to a person are described as core constructs; less important ones as peripheral.

All these constructs – whether easily verbalised or experienced as feelings, abstract or more concrete, core or peripheral – are linked together to form our 'construct system'. And it is through this system that a person develops theories about things in order to find ways of dealing with the world. Experience of events and people will cause us to modify these theories and elaborate them over time. Our sense of ourselves will change as we become involved in a wider range of activities. Learning something new will give rise to new ideas. New relationships will evoke new feelings. Validation or invalidation from others may affect our overall picture of who we are at any point.

Processes of construing

When we seek to understand another's experience we need not only to make sure that we have grasped the very personal meaning of the words used but also the non-verbal language of posture, gesture and facial expression. Especially where there are communication difficulties, attention to construing at all levels will be essential. Through it we may be able to see things through their eyes and take on both the content of their construing and, just as important, the ways in which events are experienced.

One of Kelly's most useful dimensions by which we can assess the ways in which a person construes is that of *tightness* and *looseness*. Construing something tightly implies that our predictions are clear-cut and sure: I'm going to meet someone new and will have to give him my name, therefore I will stutter and stutter badly. Loose construing, on the other hand, leaves more room for manoeuvre: I'm meeting a new person so I may have trouble with my speech. If he seems friendly, though, or if I can relax a bit it may be all right. If a client's construing is excessively tight we must bear in mind that it will be more difficult for him or her to consider alternative outcomes. If someone construes extremely loosely there may be difficulty in anticipating how things will be at all. Most of us move from tight to loose construing according to context but we may have areas of tightness that prevent us from being open to new possibilities or looseness which makes decision-making fraught with anxiety.

Another aspect of Kelly's approach that takes us beyond the content of a person's construing is the strong emphasis on the awareness of states of transition. When clients or those about them are having difficulty making sense of areas of life or of another's behaviour it can be useful to look at their feelings of unease in relation to how they experience themselves at the time. Kelly defines the generally vague states of anxiety, guilt and threat in specific terms that can help to clarify the individual's situation.

Anxiety is the awareness that we are unable to make sense of what confronts us, whether it is an event or the behaviour of another person. We cannot predict what will happen when we go for that interview or sit that exam. We don't understand why a person does what he does or says what he says. Worst of all, we can't anticipate our own behaviour or feelings in a particular circumstance. One way in which the counsellor might help to lessen the anxiety is by making situations more predictable through gaining information about what is to come. If the client can make more sense of another's behaviour through attempting to see things through that person's eyes, he or she may find things less disturbing.

Guilt is seen in terms of dislodgement of the self from how we have believed ourselves to be. Usually feelings of guilt are associated with the notion that we have done something wrong. Here the implication is of being 'out of character'. A child who has long ago accepted that he is a bad lot will experience this kind of guilt if he is praised for being good. A woman who has seen herself first and foremost as a mother may feel empty and useless, at least for a time, when the children leave home. It can be very helpful to explore such feelings with a counsellor. This may enable the person to accept them as part of the process of change.

Threat is described as the awareness of imminent comprehensive change in the construing of oneself. Awareness of the implications of impending change, such as the possible loss of a job, of a loved person who is seriously ill or of deterioration in one's own health, are obvious examples of events that could make us deeply apprehensive. Less obviously 'threatening' are such events as a coming marriage, promotion or the achievement of a longed-for goal such as fluency or weight loss. People may experience painful feelings, fears of not being able to cope, because the extent of the change in self-perception is overwhelming.

Kelly describes two contrasting ways of dealing with the awareness of transition and the discomfort this evokes. A person may adopt a hostile approach, denying that change has occurred or will occur, clinging to an old construction of things despite evidence to the contrary. Or he or she may show aggression, which in Kelly's terms is an active readiness to confront new things, to try new ways of dealing with changed circumstances or to look at another's actions in a new light. In the counselling process hostility can prove a serious block to progress and we often need to help the client to develop a more aggressive approach in the face of anxiety or threat.

These are just a few of the important concepts that are at the heart of Kelly's approach to psychological intervention, chosen for their particular relevance to work with Mark.

Special issues for hearing-impaired adolescents

Much has been written about the effects of hearing loss on the development of language in young people. Bamford and Saunders (1991) examine the descriptive research in this area and come to the conclusion that

> bearing in mind the heterogeneity of the hearing impaired child population, in terms of age, hearing loss, background, and so on, there are insufficient data to allow us yet to give a comprehensive description of the development of language in various groups . . . we are nowhere near yet fulfilling even a developmental description of the language of the hearing-impaired child.

They do, however, usefully lead us to consider both the primary cause of poor language performance because of depletion of sensory input and the associated secondary effects. These latter are concerned with the contextual aspects of language acquisition, which can be divided into processes that are external to the child and those that are internal.

External processes include 'adult–child interactions, turn-taking, adult control of the communication process in the face of reduced communicative abilities in the child'. Internal aspects refer to 'the cognitive processes and strategies brought to bear by the hearing-impaired child in the face of reduced sensory input'. As Mark's use of language was remarkably effective in the one-to-one context of our conversations and he showed little sign of cognitive delay or deficit, my concern in counselling was more with the effect of external factors on the nature of his construing.

Effects on construing of hearing impairment

I had learned from working with a number of hearing-impaired children that each one will deal with the lack of auditory input in his or her own way. One boy showed very little awareness of what he was missing and no curiosity about what people were saying unless they spoke directly to him. He was concerned that people should listen to his 'facts' (opinions) but showed little interest in exchanging views about things. A five-year-old girl watched her mother all the time and used her as her main channel of information as to what was expected of her. Mark, as we shall see, was relentless in his demands to know what was going on. The parents of a young girl who had some hearing for environmental sounds had from the beginning drawn the child's attention to objects that produced visible and tactile as well as auditory signals – the steam from a boiling kettle, for example, or the vibration in the cat's body as it purred.

Most children are sensitive to facial expression that conveys a dimension of a person's meaning, though it can mislead, as we shall see. Those who are unable to hear cannot, of course, pick up the nuances of intonation. Irony is lost on them and verbal humour generally is impoverished for them. Physical contact will express much that words cannot and those children whose families relate through touching will feel more included than those whose families are not demonstrative.

It is this aspect of the experience of being deaf that is the most crucial for many such children. Although few can express it directly unless they have become deaf after some years of hearing, there is a sense for them of being shut in, cut off from a world which they can view but of which they cannot feel fully a part. Adding to this the degree of dependency most of them have on their mothers in particular, their sense of self must be unlike that of most hearing young people. They are at once more separated from other people and more bound to them by need. Construing other people, too, will be more difficult. We are very dependent on spoken language and tones of voice in our attempts to gauge each other's moods and intentions. Where the child's own communicative abilities are impaired they are also more difficult for others to construe. All this makes for isolation.

Issues of confidentiality

In Dalton (1994) I attempt to address the complex problem of confidentiality when working with young people. Up to a point their rights must be the same as those of adults. 'Counsellors undertake to respect all that clients tell them as private, with the proviso that where they feel that clients are likely to be a danger to themselves or others through what they are doing they may, preferably with the client's knowledge, involve someone else.' Children with communication problems may present special difficulties here. If they are used to depending on others to interpret and convey their meanings and feelings they may themselves have no notion of privacy and their parents set no boundaries beyond which they will not intrude.

Clearly the counsellor, like the speech and language therapist, will need to talk to the parents if only in relation to changes that they might helpfully make. But it is important that the child is able to trust the counsellor when he or she says that something will remain private and to be helped to understand when something needs to be passed on.

The client's story

Mark's mother, Marion, came to see me a few weeks before his thirteenth birthday. She told how he had been severely deafened at the age of three as a result of meningitis. She described how hard it had been to accept that his hearing would not improve and remained angry at the 'unfairness' of the situation for the whole family. She and her husband often wondered what life would have been like if the trauma had not happened: what kind of a boy Mark would have been and how different things would have been for their daughter who was a year old when Mark became ill.

Marion had found it difficult to give adequate attention to both children in the early years and believed that she had handled the situation badly. Jealousy between the two children had become so great that the parents felt it was better to keep them apart. The girl, Rosemary, was sent to boarding school. Marion gave up her work as a medical secretary for many years and had not long returned to work part time. Both maternal and paternal grandparents had taken a great interest in Mark and the extended family as a whole seemed supportive.

I asked her what support she had had for herself outside the family. In the early years, it appeared, there had been some and the 'medical people' had done their best but there had been nothing in the way of counselling at that traumatic time. The family seemed to have looked to various associations for practical help and advice but never became involved in support groups or with other families of children with hearing impairment. She brushed aside any notion of personal help for herself. She did not need anyone to talk to – just for people to understand Mark's needs.

Although all possible help was sought for him, Marion in particular had been determined that Mark should not go to a school for the deaf. Somehow she had managed for him to have sufficient extra support to attend a small private school near home. Soon he would be taking the exams for a new and much larger school. Although he coped well academically he had always had difficulty relating to other children. He excelled in some sports but disliked team games where he could be confused. Some of the teachers at his present school found him hard to deal with but the headmistress had been his champion from the start.

Marion described Mark as lovable but 'difficult from the word go'. He had been hyperactive before his illness and losing his hearing had increased the wildness of his frustration. He hated to miss out on what was going on and continually demanded to know what people were saying and what things meant that he failed to understand. Although longing for friends he alienated other children by his impatience and constantly complained of being left out. She felt confident that he would find some work that he could do but was fearful for his future socially.

Marion had always been her son's only confidante and, although she was pleased that he could talk openly to her, she had begun to be concerned by his dependency on her alone. His father 'did his best' for him but could be very impatient and said that she spoiled him. When Marion suggested counselling for the boy to help with relationships her husband's first reaction had been negative – surely he had enough special attention? He eventually agreed, however, and Mark himself was in favour, asking that his mother should speak to me first and tell me how things were. Although I was also a speech therapist I was not expected to help him with either speech or lip-reading (although Mark asked me to pull him up if he made any mistakes). We negotiated the issues of confidentiality to be put to Mark before he came and agreed on four exploratory sessions if he felt comfortable at our first meeting.

Although Mark was to be my client the closeness of the bond between himself and his mother made it even more important than usual in working with young people that I should be aware of her constructs – about Mark, about his problem and about her own role in relation to him. That she cared for him was not in doubt and she seemed to have devoted the greater part of her time and energy to his welfare over the past ten years. She clearly found him explosive and difficult and her concern for him was tempered with exasperation. The notion of 'unfairness' seemed a core construct and anger a powerful family response to what had happened. There were hints that father resented her preoccupation with Mark and I could only wonder where the situation left his sister Rosemary. I had a sense that by now Marion no longer felt able to control things for Mark.

The hearing impairment

Marion brought with her a copy of a detailed report by an educational psychologist specialising in work with children with a hearing impairment. She recorded that he had no hearing in his right ear and that his aided threshold in his left ear was 30–55 decibels. (He used a radio link in the classroom.) His lip-reading ability was exceptional and the speech therapy he had from early on resulted in articulation and voice quality within normal range. His language skills, both comprehension and expression, were within average limits for his age but there were gaps in his vocabulary and knowledge because of his inability to use conversational context fully. The need for him to concentrate was very demanding and he would inevitably 'switch off' sometimes, possibly missing key points in a lesson or longer conversation. She was very impressed by his determination and academic achievements in the face of such impairment.

The first meeting

When he came with his mother and we spoke together for a short time before moving to another room I was struck by two things: by his intensity as he watched us both, not wanting to miss anything that was said, and by the way his mother shouted, the effort distorting her face into harshness. They seemed irritable with each other, although he was polite and charming to me.

When we left his mother I asked him what he felt he might need my help with and he said at once 'other people'. He didn't get on with people at school. In fact he had only one friend – otherwise there was just his family. When I tried to explore what might go wrong he said 'I'm here for you to tell me what's wrong with them!' What did he think was wrong with them? They 'hadn't a clue', had no idea what it was like to be deaf. They talked about him, wouldn't let him join in things. I asked him whether he had ever tried to tell any of them what it was like or what he could and could not do? He shrugged and said 'Only James – he's all right'. He told me about school. The teachers were OK and he could do most of the work. Sometimes, though, he missed out on what the homework was about and got into trouble. It wasn't really fair. He liked English and art and squash and had just got a new computer. He inspected mine and decided that it wasn't bad. He wanted to see whether the printer was as good as his and I promised he could try it next time.

When we got on to his family he said that his sister was OK. He didn't really see much of her. He spoke warmly of his maternal grandparents and said that they lived in a huge house in Suffolk. It was great. He loved going there. His father was busy most of the time. They argued a lot but he was quite kind really. Mum was all right but she kept on at him about his room. I remembered how loudly his mother had spoken while she was with us and asked him whether he could hear my voice. He said no, but it didn't matter. He could even read what I said if I turned sideways. Could he hear his mother's voice? Sort of. But not what she was saying.

I asked him whether he knew any other people with a hearing problem and he said 'not really'. He did not want to mix with them because they would 'pull him down'. If he had gone to a school for the deaf he wouldn't have had to work so hard but he wouldn't have got anywhere. People didn't expect anything of you. It seemed likely that much of this was his mother's view, but he had clearly taken it on board.

By the end of the session I had heard something of Mark's current life and gained the impression of an intelligent, enthusiastic, impatient boy, with a short fuse and a sense of humour. When I spoke of confidentiality he grinned and said 'You mean, my secret is safe with you?' He shared his mother's sense of the unfairness of things. He told how he had arrived late at the squash courts the evening before, they had started without him and he found himself without a partner. His belief that people talked about him and deliberately left him out further set him apart from others. He clearly felt that everyone should understand his experience and it would undoubtedly be important to help him to question this view and find a way of communicating aspects of his situation.

He readily agreed to four sessions to explore things and seemed to like the idea of a grid. I asked him to write a character sketch of himself for next time and he left reminding me of my promise to let him try the computer.

Exploring Mark's view of himself and his world

The two best-known means in PCP of exploring the client's world are the self-characterisation and repertory grid technique. First people are asked to write a character sketch of themselves in the third person – as if through the eyes of an intimate and sympathetic friend. Next, a sample of constructs is elicited from comparing and contrasting a range of elements (in most cases significant people in the client's life) and then rating or rank ordering them according to where they see them on a chosen scale (see Table 2.1).

The self-characterisation and a story

Like many young people Mark ignored the use of the third person and it would probably have been difficult for him to imagine an intimate friend. The following sketch is short and, at first sight, not very revealing:

> I am 12 years old and I am in form five of . . . School. I am deaf and I live in . . .. My interests and hobbies are art and all sports except rugby. I am especially good at squash and model making. I am also very interested in electronics and technical equipment. I already have a remote control plane and car. I also have a keen interest in computers and robots. When I leave . . . I go to . . . School and hope to do good art and play squash well. I am not sure what I want to do when I grow up but I hope to study at engineering and computers or maybe art. I have a sister called Rosemary and I am having a lot of problems with my friends. I am impatient and have a bad temper.

Since no instructions are given as to the content of a self-characterisation it is assumed that the person will write about what is important to him or her. Boys of this age often refer to possessions and it is not unusual to list what they are 'good at'. It is interesting, knowing that the two children had to be separated, that he refers to his sister and the 'friends' he is having problems within the same sentence. His final 'I am impatient and have a bad temper' sounds like family labelling. This is very much a boy on his own.

Mark gave me the sketch saying that it wasn't very good. He'd forgotten all about it until that morning. At the same time he handed me a short story he had written, where he shows a very different side of himself. Called 'The Face at the Window' it tells how the author has a big fight with one of his class-mates. He is driven home 'bruised and bleeding' and is unable to do his homework for thinking about it. He looks at the window and sees a face in it. It is the boy he fought. This happens four times and each time the face has a different expression on it: first 'fierce and unhappy', second 'almost hidden by a black eye', third 'badly bruised' and fourth 'crying'. He is very shaken by this experience and thinks about it for a long time. He realises the meaning of the sequence of faces: 'the first – revenge, the second – hurt, the third – very badly hurt, the last – retreat'. When he goes to school the next day the boy seems to be very friendly, apologising. He tries to apologise too. That evening he sees two faces in the window – that of himself and the boy 'smiling and happy'.

As Mark gave the story to me rather shyly and went straight over to the computer I simply read it and thanked him without asking him any questions at that time. It did seem, though, that he was aware of, even wanting, alternatives to strife and revenge. His awareness of the suffering of the other boy contrasts strongly with his dismissive attitude to most of his peers. Although I have found young people's self-characterisations useful, imaginative writing such as this can often touch on feelings that they would not otherwise express. A little later on Mark drew a picture of his grandparents' house that had great freedom and flow about it. Getting young people to invent stories as well as to draw can access construing at deeper levels of awareness and help them to loosen. The work of Ravenette is full of ideas for this kind of indirect access (for example, Ravenette 1977, 1980).

The rated grid

When eliciting constructs for a grid it is most usual to ask adults to say in what important way two people are alike and thereby different from a third. Younger people are often asked to compare just two people or even to say what is important about one, the opposite being found through asking how they would describe someone 'really very different from that'. Table 2.1 (page 46) shows constructs elicited from Mark by a combination of the last two methods with their ratings on a nine-point scale.

Mark chose his family as elements, two of his teachers and the rest were boys he had known for a long time, James being his one 'real friend'. He also agreed to include 'me now' and 'me as I'd like to be' so that we could see where he might want to be different. Looking down the columns of the two selves we can see that he rates himself positively overall but there are some changes he would like. The two major ones are from being not at all liked to being liked and, at the very extremes, from having great problems with friends to having no problems with them. He would also like to be more patient, but not excessively so (he explained that he wouldn't know himself if he were too patient). I needed to know what he meant by 'not being noticed' as he saw himself now and it linked with his sense of being ignored. His rating of himself as he would like to be at the mid-point here, however, meant that he didn't want to be noticed for the wrong reason, namely because he was deaf. Wanting to be less 'sensible' was to do with being able to take life less seriously. He could not explain exactly what 'reacts to others' reactions' meant but it seemed to be something of a family construct to do with minding what other people were thinking.

He rated his parents and teachers positively on the whole. Not so his sister. And 'Thomas' is clearly one of the 'friends' he has trouble with, scoring many '1's and '9's. He had originally also wanted to include 'me as I seem' but found it difficult to rate. He felt sure that he was different inside from how he appeared to others, but it was

Table 2.1: The raw data of Mark's repertory grid

Ratings are on a scale of 1 to 9

1 ← → 9

Element	1	2	3	4	5	6	7	8	9	10	11	12	13	14	15
Harry	4	5	3	5	7	3	2	1	2	1	3	5	7	1	6
Thomas	4	8	—	8	9	1	9	1	1	1	9	1	9	1	5
Robert B	8	2	8	3	3	5	4	8	7	9	3	8	1	5	8
James	3	3	1	9	4	4	3	2	8	2	9	1	8	2	5
Bridget	9	2	9	—	8	8	—	9	—	7	1	8	2	1	—
Robert L	7	5	4	3	4	8	8	8	2	1	1	2	9	5	8
Mr Tomes	5	—	6	5	6	8	1	9	3	7	1	7	5	1	—
As I'd like to be	1	1	9	1	5	6	1	7	3	—	1	6	1	5	9
John	8	9	7	5	7	1	8	2	5	1	8	3	9	1	8
Callum	3	1	9	3	5	5	2	5	2	7	6	7	1	5	7
Mr Parker	2	3	8	—	6	7	1	9	3	8	1	7	5	1	—
Daniel	2	5	6	3	7	3	2	5	4	2	5	5	3	5	7
Me now	1	1	8	7	5	3	1	5	3	—	2	8	1	7	1
Rosemary	7	3	5	—	7	5	5	4	3	3	5	3	6	1	5
Dad	3	2	8	1	4	2	7	9	2	7	2	4	2	5	9
Mum	5	1	9	1	5	5	9	8	2	7	4	5	2	5	9

Constructs:

1. Same interest as me/different interests
2. Helpful/unhelpful
3. Joking too much and teasing/doesn't tease
4. Liked/not liked
5. Shy/show off
6. Impatient/patient
7. Keen on sport/inactive
8. Lazy/works hard
9. Reacts to others' reactions/ignores others' reactions
10. Makes me embarrassed/doesn't make me embarrassed
11. Clever/stupid
12. Silly/sensible
13. Friendly/unfriendly
14. People notice you/people don't notice you
15. Has problems with friends/doesn't have problems with friends

perhaps too threatening to specify, particularly as he saw himself as 'not liked'. We were to work on this later.

The computer analysis clusters the constructs and elements according to their ratings, drawing together those that correlate significantly, either positively or negatively. The first component of the constructs (Figure 2.1) shows his preoccupation with interrelationship. In his experience people who are 'helpful', very important to him, are also friendly, sensible, don't tease or embarrass and so on. The first component of the elements (Figure 2.2) he described as the 'good' people: both parents, a cousin, Bridget, the two teachers, James and two other friends, whom he had known for a long time. Thomas and John, being negatively correlated, stand in contrast as the raw data would suggest. In another component these two boys are grouped with his sister Rosemary.

Mark expressed himself as satisfied with the outcome of the grid and we agreed that it clarified at least one main area for us to work on: the effect he might have on others by the way he behaved towards them. Although not about to go back on his sense of other people's unfairness towards him he was willing to try to gauge the part he played in interractions.

The transitive diagnosis

The purpose of a transitive diagnosis in PCP terms is to clarify aspects of a client's construing that need to be taken into account

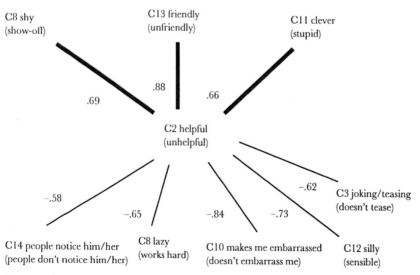

Figure 2.1: The first component of the constructs.

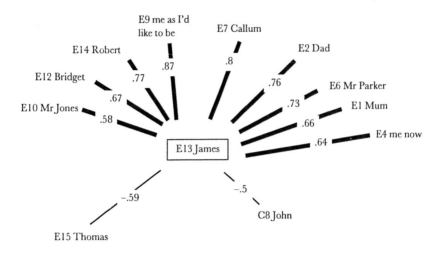

Figure 2.2: The first component of the elements in Mark's grid.

when working for change. Mark's construing of people at least was clearly tight. This is not only shown by the number of high correlations in the grid and the methodical listing of abilities and possessions in the self-characterisation but also came across strongly in conversation: almost all boys are clueless, teachers are OK, nothing is expected of deaf people.

   With such pre-emptive construing we often find hostility – proving your point at all costs. The one or two instances of unfairness which Mark had described suggested that people's behaviour simply fulfilled his firm predictions of them. The short story, however, does show an easing of hostility and the drawing of his grandparents' house has an impressionistic feel to it, showing that in some contexts at least he can construe more loosely. His mother had clearly begun to be concerned about Mark's dependence on her. Underlying his difficulty in relating to people outside the family and the one or two people he had known for a long time there seemed to be a serious problem of undispersed dependencies (Kelly 1955/1991, pp.913–20). He could turn to other adults, such as teachers, for practical help but was unable to trust people with his needs and feelings – especially his peers.

Initial aims

Since relationships with other young people was Mark's own area of greatest concern, these clearly had to be our priority. The following aspects seemed important:

- Mark had little idea of how people might see him and what effect his attitude towards others might have on them;
- he seemed to feel that people should just 'know' how things were for him but had made little attempt to communicate his experience to others;
- he showed little interest in other people's experience and assumed that life was easy for everyone else.

Mark's preoccupation with himself was entirely understandable but was clearly an obstacle to developing relationships. He therefore needed:

- to be more aware of how his behaviour might be construed by others;
- to finds ways of communicating his situation and his needs to others which were compatible with his sense of himself;
- to learn to 'read' other people more effectively, despite his lack of so important a dimension of potential understanding, and consider their behaviour, moods etc. other than as they related to himself.

Movement in these areas would clearly involve some loosening of his constructions of others and of his place amongst them. A reduction in hostility was essential and he needed to develop the wider range of dependencies appropriate to a young person in order to enjoy a fuller life. When I explained these aims to Mark (in somewhat less formal language) he felt that the first and second would probably help, groaning at the third – he said that his father was always on at him about this – 'being too wrapped up in himself'. I emphasised how hard it was to make sense of people when you had only what you saw to go by and he agreed to see what we could do about it.

The process of counselling over a six-month period

We first met in early January and worked together on a weekly basis, with breaks for Easter and during the two half-terms until mid-July. To begin with Mark came armed with a list of grievances about the behaviour of other boys towards him during the past week. He found it difficult at first to focus on his part in any exchange and needed some convincing that I was not asking him to shift the blame on to himself instead. As he had implied, I was supposed to be helping him change them. The notion that he was the only one he could change was a hard one for him to accept.

Loosening the construing of events and people

I used his detailed accounts of various incidents to analyse them in terms of (a) what the other person might be thinking, feeling, intending and (b) how he might come across in the exchange. The first sign of loosening came when he began to imagine a range of alternatives. On one occasion, for example, he had come into the classroom and found Harry talking to another boy. They had stopped when Mark entered and looked 'embarrassed'. His immediate assumption was that they were talking about him and he'd felt very annoyed and stomped out again. What would they have thought of that? That he was in a bad temper.

How else could it have been? He supposed they could have been talking about something they'd done wrong and didn't want anyone to know. Some 'rude pictures' were being passed round and it might have been that. How else could he have behaved? Ignored it. Asked them what was going on. Played it cool.

In the course of such explorations it emerged that Mark longed to be friendly but, in his anxiety to understand, probably often looked 'frowny' and cross. He drew an amusing picture of himself like this, then another all smiles with a halo. He felt he couldn't be friendly when he didn't know what to say to people. The others talked a lot about television programmes they'd seen, for example. He found most of them difficult to follow so couldn't join in. How else did people show that they were friendly? They smiled, they asked people about their things, they did something helpful. So he did have some ideas.

Questioning his immediate negative assumptions did seem to put something of a break on his impulsive responses. Then he came with a finding of his own: someone could be 'horrible' one minute and kind the next. He had realised that his own mood could swing but had found it difficult to accept that others were inconsistent too. He was also able to ponder whether another boy's bad mood need have anything at all to do with him. Even James could be 'shirty' when he was beaten at squash.

Communicating his needs to others

It was more difficult for him to reconstrue his own behaviour and the effect it might have on others and it seemed likely that he could make more inroads here when he went to the new school with a new group of people. The boys in his class had already decided that he was prickly and 'unfriendly' but it did seem to make a difference when at last he felt able to explain something of the implications of his hearing loss to some of them. He arrived one day saying that he had 'confided' in a boy with whom he was working on a computer. At first the boy took over and seemed to assume that Mark couldn't cope. For once he didn't walk off but explained what he could do and where the boy could help him by making sure that he didn't miss the instructions. His companion was apparently very interested and asked him more about his deafness. Someone next to them was listening and Mark didn't mind!

At about the same time he met a boy with a severe stammer who was to go to the school he hoped to get into. We were able to use this difficulty to find some parallels with Mark's situation. Until the boy told him what his experience was like Mark had no idea how he felt or how difficult many situations could be for him. Mark had assumed he was 'not very bright' at first but as he did well in most subjects this clearly wasn't so. Most significantly, when the boy stammered he looked tense and angry, although he was quite good-natured and friendly. This, in particular, linked with Mark's appearance when he was struggling to understand what was going on.

Developing sociality: construing others' construing

As Mark took more than his usual interest in this new friend, Roger, I used him as someone he could try to 'read' in more depth. I asked him to write a self-characterisation of him as if he were Roger. He hadn't known him long but he was able to guess that he saw himself as 'quite bright', with a 'clever Dad', a big house, 'good-tempered' and 'strong', with a problem with his speech which people were quite good about. It was a start.

When he referred to something Roger or one of the others had said or done I often asked him what he thought they were thinking and feeling. He caught onto this and got there before me once or twice. For example, when he described a teacher losing his temper with the class he added: 'He was feeling really fed up and thinking "What have I done to deserve this?"' Touché! He really had begun to be more interested in what was going on in others.

Although Mark continued to have difficulty with some people at school he noticeably brought more news of 'good things' as time went on. Some of these were to do with successes at squash or in art, others with relationships. He seemed to be spending time with a somewhat wider range of people and to be more willing to construe them as separate from himself. His sister had been home for the Easter holidays and he was quite dismissive when I asked how they had got on. I was tempted to pursue this area further but recognised that it was very deep and fraught with hazards. We had enough to do already.

Meeting with mother

Mark said at the end of the first session after Easter that his mother would like to talk to me. I asked him how he felt about that and he said 'fine'. She was apparently worried about the exams and the interview for the new school. He 'wasn't bothered'. He'd be all right. He hoped I'd be telling her to stop pushing him about work. Life was 'one long test'.

Marion had kept to her resolve not to intervene in the counselling unless she was really concerned about something, which was good, but this meant that I had missed the build-up of her anxiety about his work. She was clearly very fraught and angry with Mark for not working harder. He had referred to arguments about it occasionally but shrugged them off. She felt that he was getting on better with other children and was on the whole calmer but this seemed less important to her at the moment than the possibility of his failing. She had worked so hard over the years to make sure he could achieve the utmost and she dreaded having to start all over again planning a future for him if he didn't get into the school of their choice. I was full of admiration for all that Marion had done for Mark but was struck once again by the intensity of her feeling for him and the pressure she put on herself and, inevitably, on him. When we looked at various aspects of this important stage in their lives Marion felt that he would do well in the interview as long as the others concerned had understood what he needed from them in terms of their communication and attitude towards him. So far, she acknowledged, she had been able to make things clear to others and they had given him every chance, but would he get his revision organised properly and do enough? It emerged that she 'had to push him every night' to do his homework and check on him that he had the right books and so forth. It was wearing her out.

I asked what part father played in all this and it appeared that he sat back and let them get on with it, although when he was involved Mark took more notice of him. After some discussion she agreed that it might help for father to take more of the responsibility for helping Mark to organise himself. He did need the help but neither of them needed the constant battle. We agreed that it wasn't my role to push him over work but I said that it would be important for me to explore any anxieties he had about the exams, the interview and the impending change to a new and larger school.

The threat of change

Marion had undoubtedly told Mark something of our conversation and he weighed straight in with complaints about her nagging. I asked him why he thought she did this and he said first that she always did, about everything, and then acknowledged that she was worried in case he failed the exams. This enabled me to focus on his feelings about them. He shifted from the bravado of the week before about not being bothered and spoke of his real difficulty in concentrating for long periods when he really wanted to be doing something else and his fear that he wouldn't do enough revision. When could he concentrate? When he was drawing and painting, playing squash, working something out on the computer. He could go on for hours. Why was this? Because he wanted to achieve something important. How important was it for him to get into this particular school? Very. He couldn't imagine going anywhere else. It would be a disaster.

It had seemed from Marion that the one alternative was far from attractive to Mark and his parents: there would be nothing like the back-up he needed, he would have much further to go and the academic standards were poor. There was no local provision for hearing-impaired pupils and, anyway, they had ruled that out long ago.

Was it possible for him to approach revision in the same way as he approached the things he liked to do? Seeing the 'grind' as a means to an end, the achievement he so badly wanted? Could he in some way reduce the battle between himself and his mother by putting some structure on his work and sticking to it? Where did he need help and where was it all down to him? What he seemed to need most of all was a coherent plan: to get himself organised before he started, making sure he had the right books and notes (others could help here) and then to set himself specific times to work, with breaks, and follow things through as he did with his drawing. Much of his anxiety was around feeling 'muddled' and disorganised and Dad was apparently good at organising.

The dependency issue

This brought us back to the battle with mother. Mark was evidently experiencing the resentment of dependency on her that would be expected in most adolescents but they were locked in by his special needs. Whether or not she 'nagged' him more than other mothers, she clearly needed to be there for him more than most mothers of boys of his age and perhaps found it particularly hard to let go when she might. For his part he knew only too well how much he relied on her and found it undermining. Looking at his day-to-day life we found many areas in which he went his own way without 'interference' and some where he could fend for himself but waited for mother to sort things out. For example, although he had a few more friends now he left it to her to plan out-of-school meetings with them. If he was unhappy about something to do with a teacher she always spoke for him. I asked him whether he felt able to approach members of the staff with a problem and he said 'yes'.

At a deeper level it emerged that he had always told her everything. She knew everything that was in his mind. Did she question him? No. He just always had told her. Did he tell his father everything? No. Some things were private. There was no way I was going to urge him to keep 'secrets' from his mother but we talked from time to time about thoughts and feelings that were what he called 'inner things' and 'news' and ideas that were good to share. Mother didn't always understand his inner things, was impatient with them, and maybe nobody could.

Kelly (1955/1991 pp.313–15) produced a situational resources repertory test, usually referred to as a dependency grid, to look at the people to whom we turn for various purposes in particular circumstances. Without actually setting one up, I used this principle to explore with him how he currently dispersed his dependencies. As expected, he would turn to his mother for almost everything but he was able to imagine, for example, talking to James about a girl he liked; sharing his thoughts about art with his grandfather who also painted. He had avoided discussing many things with people outside the family in case he lost track but could ask more people to make sure he could see their faces now that he recognised that they genuinely wouldn't think of it unless he did. Above all, it seemed clear that he could do more for himself if he chose and if mother didn't automatically step in. He agreed to talk about this with her when there was a specific example.

Testing times

In the period leading up to the examinations and the interview Mark's moods inevitably swung from determination, to irritability, to frenzy. He did seem to be better organised with his father's help and a certain solidarity sprang up between himself and a few friends over their time of trial but there were frequent explosions with his mother and some trouble at school where his impatience spilled over at some 'unfairness' to do with his misunderstanding some work and being marked down for it. He thumped his desk and bruised his wrist badly. This sobered him somewhat and he later apologised to the teacher with no prompting from anyone.

The interview took place just before the exams and he acquitted himself well. 'Turned on the charm' according to Marion and, as so often, had them rooting for him. He still wanted to come to talk right up to the exams, although the subject of our discourse was understandably narrow. He brought some of the work he had done for his art project and I was again struck by the freedom and imagination of his painting. The examinations came and went and we waited for the results. He passed.

Preparing for the future

As there were only a few weeks left before the family was due to go away on holiday I clarified some final aims with Mark to round off the counselling series. We would:

- look back at our initial aims and see how far he had made changes;
- try to anticipate the implications of the changes that were to come;
- we also needed to agree on the nature of any further contact between us.

Assessing change

As an alternative to re-rating his grid we went through the ratings of 'me now' and 'me as I'd like to be' to see whether he felt there had been any movement on the constructs where there had been a marked difference in rating (see Figure 2.1):

- for 'liked' versus 'not liked' he thought he might be about in the middle now as some people seemed friendlier towards him;
- he was perhaps a bit more 'patient' rather than 'impatient' over some things, but he could still get really mad sometimes;
- he pondered over 'people notice you' versus 'people don't notice you' and it emerged that the meaning of the construct had changed for him. Earlier he had felt unnoticed because he was left out and put himself as wanting to be in the middle

because although he wanted attention he didn't want to be noticed for his deafness. Now he would put himself as '3' for being noticed as he had done well and felt more involved in things and would like to be '1' – 'a star';

- he still saw himself as having problems with friends but he rated this as '4' rather than '1'.

Mark seemed quite pleased with this.

The first aim we had listed was to be more aware of how his behaviour might be seen by others and the second to find ways of communicating his situation and his needs to them. We agreed that being more communicative had led to fewer misunderstandings and that he had been able to show that he was the 'friendly' person he knew himself to be to some people at least. As for the third aim, he reckoned that he had become something of a 'psychologist' in his efforts to read other people and 'get into their minds'!

From a PCP point of view all this had involved some loosening and some lessening of hostility. He was less inclined to take everything personally and as 'against' him. It was difficult to tell how far the spreading of his dependencies had developed. He was certainly sharing more with others outside the family and taking more responsibility for things himself but there was no doubt that his mother was still the key figure in his life.

Looking forward

It was now early July and almost time for a holiday in France. Mark was very excited about it and not very interested in anticipating how things would be at the new school. We agreed, therefore – with his parents' consent – that we should meet again nearer the time to discuss things. Marion, too, said that she would like to meet after their holiday and that a teacher especially assigned to support Mark wanted to come to see me. Mark was quite happy for me to say what I liked to her.

The teacher was a young woman who was clearly feeling her responsibility keenly. She had found Marion full of practical advice for which she was grateful but she was clearly very anxious as to how Mark would cope, knowing the demands of a large and very active school. She had construed him as charming and lively but impulsive and disorganised. We agreed that her major role would be to help him work out a system for organising himself in new surroundings and to make sure that he understood what was expected of him. She thought she might enlist the help of various boys in the different 'sets' in which he would work to check that he was clear about homework, for instance. (I suggested that Mark be involved in choosing who might be approached and that she make sure that he felt comfortable about it.) We agreed to keep in contact.

I met Marion again after their holiday and she was clearly very apprehensive. Having achieved one goal she now saw years of worry ahead of her, having to make sure that Mark kept his head above water. She was encouraged by what I told her of my meeting with the teacher and resolved to continue to leave more to her husband in the way of helping Mark to organise things at home. They had had a good holiday but she felt that Rosemary had become 'remote' and she was concerned about her. Her husband, it seemed, was tired of her worrying. She began to say something about her feelings of 'guilt' but swiftly changed the subject. I referred again to the possibility of her seeing someone for herself and, this time, she said that she would think about it.

Mark, when he came, was full of excitement and all decked out in his school uniform to show it to me. There was no way we could have a solemn conversation about how he was going to cope but we did touch on some of the important issues about relating to new people. We listed what seemed to be the key points: he would set about 'reading' people and try to put himself in their shoes (he felt he'd become something of an expert at this with some people on holiday); he would learn about their things; he would tell them about himself if they seemed friendly and interested.

He guessed that he wouldn't have time for regular meetings with me but wanted to know that he could come 'if something cropped up'. Although his special teacher wasn't a counsellor she would be there for him if he needed to talk about things that worried him. At the end of the session he took a card out of his satchel which he had made himself. On the front was a picture of the house where they had stayed in France. Inside he had illustrated some of his constructs with cartoon faces: friendly/unfriendly, patient/impatient, lazy/works hard, clever/stupid.

Reflections

There were a number of issues I could have addressed with Mark or his mother but chose not to because of the limited time we were likely to have. At our first meeting it was clear that Marion and her husband did not want Mark to be part of 'the deaf culture'. I could perhaps have explored this with her further but I simply accepted the decision that she and her husband had made many years earlier. I was very concerned about the situation with their daughter and full of questions about the implications for all the members of the family. Sooner or later I would hope that some change could be effected in relationships between them, but this was not the time and the father and Rosemary herself would have to be involved.

I have often worked with a parent and child as a couple and could have done so in this case. There was obviously a good deal of tension and strife between Mark and his mother, which could perhaps have been eased by working together, but Marion's dismissal of any thoughts of counselling for herself seemed to rule this out. I predicted, rightly or wrongly, that the area that both of them presented as that of greatest frustration for him, his relationships with his peers, would become swamped if we focused on the relationship between the two of them. Added to this it seemed appropriate, given his extreme dependency on her, that the sessions should be his alone, where he could try to deal with what troubled him for himself.

One young person's experience of hearing loss

I had read about the effects of hearing loss on language development and cognitive functioning. I had understood something of the secondary effects that relate to the contextual aspects of language acquisition but it was only from Mark himself that I learned something of the very personal experience of living without the faculty of hearing. For him, the important losses were to do with missing out on what was going on, being unable fully to join with others in discussing shared events, not being able to judge when an action, a look, a comment referred to him.

Although his sense of his own worth was in many ways strong, he had grave doubts about being valued by others, which I hope were lessened through our work. He looked forward to the future in terms of a career with reasonable confidence but on the rare occasions when he referred to girls, whom he was obviously beginning to find attractive, he clearly found it difficult to imagine relating closely with them. He could feel a real sense of achievement when he was drawing or painting or working at the computer but these were solitary pursuits. He looked forward to it when he was invited to parties but usually came away dissatisfied because he'd been confused and distracted instead of joining in the fun he saw that others were having.

I learned a lot from working with Mark and hope that our conversations made a difference to him as they did to me. I admired his courage and felt for his frustration. He came to see me once or twice after he began at the new school. He had made one or two good friends and found people generally friendly and helpful. He found the work hard and it sometimes got on top of him but on the whole he 'managed'. On his last visit he told me that he had won a prize in art and he was being encouraged by the art master to think of specialising. I hope he did.

Chapter 3
Fran: understanding and treating psychogenic dysphonia from a cognitive-behavioural perspective

PETER BUTCHER AND LESLEY CAVALLI

Introduction – the case history – the voice therapy programme – psychological assessment and treatment – edited transcript of psychological treatment sessions – post-treatment assessment – conclusions.

Introduction

Patients with psychogenic voice change usually gain significant benefit from a standard course of voice therapy (Carding and Horsley 1992). However, many of these patients leave the therapist with a feeling that there are underlying causes of a psychological nature that have not been resolved by the patient or addressed by the voice therapist and a concern that these may create future problems or a predisposition to relapse. There is also a small number of patients who fail to show improvements with voice therapy techniques without early psychological intervention.

Setting aside those patients whose non-organic voice disorder occurs through vocal misuse or through periodic or habitual patterns of vocal abuse, we are left with a population that consistently shows common features. The typical patient with psychogenic dysphonia/aphonia is female (Aronson et al. 1966; Barton 1960; Brodnitz 1969; Butcher et al. 1987; House and Andrews 1987).

Except for a very small percentage who can be confidently diagnosed as having all the features of hysterical conversion disorder, they do not appear to have any serious psychological disturbance (Aronson et al. 1966; Aronson 1990; Butcher et al. 1987; House and Andrews 1987). Almost all are suffering from anxiety that is associated with stressful, unresolved long-term or recent life events (Aronson 1990; Butcher et al. 1987; House and Andrews 1988; Greene and Mathieson 1989). These stresses are mostly caused by marital, family and interpersonal relationship difficulties (Brodnitz 1969; Butcher et al. 1987; House and Andrews 1988). While life stress and interpersonal difficulties are commonly associated with anxiety symptoms, patients with psychogenic voice disorders almost invariably show tendencies that distinguish them from other groups of anxiety disorder patients. These tendencies include taking the main burden of responsibility within the family; feeling powerless about making personal change or altering their situation; having difficulty with assertiveness or expressing inner feelings; suppressing anger and frustration and converting these emotions into musculoskeletal tension (Aronson 1990; Butcher et al. 1987; Butcher 1995; House and Andrews 1987, 1988).

Considering the features described above, it is easy to see why these individuals might be prone to voice loss/change. They are not only more stressed and carrying more responsibilities than most but caught in troubled relationships where they feel helpless and angry because they cannot, or do not, express their feelings. When emotional conflicts and the resulting musculoskeletal tension become focused around the main organ of expression, it is hardly surprising that the voice suffers.

Viewing psychogenic voice loss from this perspective, we can now consider in what ways it differs from the interpretation of non-organic voice loss contained in Freud's general theory of hysterical conversion disorder (Freud 1896/1962; Barsky 1989).

Sigmund Freud's hysterical conversion theory was first proposed in 1896. It was later revised with developments in psychoanalytic theory. In its final form the theory states that a hysterical conversion reaction occurs when particular situations cause conflicts over expressing sexual or aggressive feelings and these impulses are repressed. During this process, the sexual/aggressive energies are converted into physical symptoms that reflect or symbolise the nature of the inner conflict. For example, loss of movement and feeling in the hand and arm might be caused by repressed and converted anxieties over either erotically touching or striking another person. As the impulse is repressed, the person remains blissfully unaware of his or her true wishes and any inner conflict this might create. Thus, a primary gain for the person suffering from a conversion disorder would be that the condition controls the forbidden impulse and repression removes any sense of subjective distress or conflict. Other, secondary gains might also exist as a consequence of the condition. For example, 'being ill' elicits sympathetic, loving or caring behaviour from others.

Over a hundred years after Freud described how psychological conflict could be converted into physical illness, his concept still provides a valuable way of understanding psychogenic forms of voice loss. However, while the general principles of the model continue to be valuable, its limitations should be noted when considering psychogenic dysphonia/aphonia (see Butcher 1995). Based on the research described above and their clinical experience, Butcher and Elias (1995) propose that there are two distinct types of psychogenic voice disorder. The first and, fortunately, rarer type fits all the criteria suggested by Freud's hysterical conversion model. Sexual conflict may be a feature (although it is likely that conflict over aggression is much more common). Individuals use repression as the main means of coping with their conflict and the unconscious conflict is converted into physical symptoms that, outwardly, symbolise the nature of the conflict. The repression may be recognisable in patients' lack of concern about their symptoms, their denial of internal or external stresses or their casual dismissal of psychological interpretations. Our attempts to treat a small number of these patients with cognitive-behavioural therapy have not been encouraging and we are of the view that alternative therapeutic approaches would probably not produce a better outcome. Thus, this population has a poor prognosis for long-term resolution of symptoms, although voice therapy may be rapidly effective in producing a 'quick fix'. The repression, denial and lack of concern make treatment difficult. There are primary as well as secondary gains that maintain the condition and there is low motivation for change because these provide sufficient reinforcement to maintain the status quo.

The second, more common, type of psychogenic voice disorder may share some of the features of hysterical conversion disorder: a predisposition to have psychological problems because of personality type, early childhood traumas, family/social taboos around expressing impulses or feelings, life experiences that increase feelings of powerlessness or lower self-esteem, and so on. They have also been exposed to a recent life event or conflict over voicing their feelings and this emotional state has been converted into physical tension which is focused on the site of the conflict – the larynx. However, here the similarity ends. Instead of using repression, this population uses suppression as a coping mechanism. In other words, these individuals consciously inhibit expressing their feelings. This means that they control the impulse but continue to experience the anxiety produced by the inner turmoil. The plus side, therapeutically, is that the conflicts are 'near the surface' and more easily accessible to the patient and therapist. While there may be some primary gains (for example, avoiding the feared consequences of expressing feelings or views), the patient cannot escape the anxiety created by the conflict. The conversion of the conflicts into a physical disorder causes additional anxieties and any secondary gains rarely provide significant compensation. Therapeutically, this is another plus. This population is highly motivated to get better because suppression, inhibition and conversion of the emotional distress into a physical problem have not resolved the external conflict or the anxiety.

Since the early 1980s we have been interested in treating psychogenic voice loss with a combination of voice therapy and cognitive-behaviour therapy (Butcher and Elias 1983; Butcher et al. 1987; Butcher et al. 1993; Elias et al. 1989). Our assumption is that the voice therapy provides the patient with skills in better use of the voice while cognitive-behaviour therapy (CBT) tackles the psychological processes underlying the disorder and provides remedial strategies. We have also assumed that once a voice therapist becomes familiar with CBT techniques he or she will offer more effective treatment programmes.

Cognitive-behaviour therapy is an established, well-researched and brief treatment for a wide range of psychological disorders. Wilson et al. (1989); Hawton et al. (1989); Blackburn and Twaddle (1996); Stern and Drummond (1991) and Scott et al. (1989) provide helpful introductions to cognitive-behavioural assessment and treatment approaches. Butcher et al. (1993) give detailed descriptions of the various ways in which CBT can be applied in the treatment of psychogenic voice disorder. A knowledge of CBT requires, for example, familiarity with how to assess thinking processes, highlight and change dysfunctional thoughts, teach *in vivo* anxiety management strategies, assess and treat depressive symptoms caused by stress and the ability to offer communication or assertiveness training and life management skills training (Butcher 1994). This being said, we have often found that psychogenic voice patients frequently respond to straightforward counselling focused on the core areas of difficulty – problematic relationships, carrying the main burden of family responsibility, inhibited expression of feelings – and need little or minimal prompting or guidance in setting their own targets for change. Thus, they can be a rewarding group to work with and, in the main, not too difficult for the voice therapist who is learning to apply psychological techniques as part of treatment.

The case we have chosen illustrates the core psychological problems underlying a typical psychogenic voice disorder. The patient is also typical in being highly motivated and benefiting from a combination of voice therapy and psychological intervention.

The case history

Fran presented at the joint ear-nose-and-throat (ENT)/speech therapy voice clinic with a two-month history of fluctuating voice change and a persistent sensation of a lump in her throat accompanied by dryness. The first impressions were that of a friendly, talkative but anxious person, in her early forties, with rapid press of speech and overall tense body posture. The following history and assessment findings resulted in a diagnosis of psychogenic dysphonia with musculoskeletal tension (Aronson 1990).

Fran's medical history revealed that she was generally fit and well with normal respiratory, endocrine, neurological and digestive systems. Of interest was the fact that she had been investigated for chest pains by the same hospital four months previously but no organic cause for her difficulties had been identified. A suggestion of anxiety related symptoms had been made to her by her doctor at this point but had not been explored further. Fran was no longer experiencing chest pains at the time of her investigations for voice difficulties.

Ear-nose-and-throat examination with laryngoscopy and stroboscopy, which offers detailed images of the anatomy and function of the larynx and vocal tract, indicated no evidence of pathology. Movement of the laryngeal structures and their associated muscles suggested mild hyperfunctional behaviours during phonation. The examination was well tolerated by Fran. A sensation of a lump in the throat, in the absence of any pathological changes, is also known as globus and occurs frequently in patients experiencing psychogenic voice changes. Greene and Mathieson (1989) note that patients with globus usually appear to have their emotions under careful control and are reluctant to express feelings. In many instances their approach to life is stoic and they continue to carry out their family and work commitments in spite of real emotional and practical difficulties. They regard the need for support from family and friends as a sign of weakness and yet there is pride in providing support for others even if at times, it is accompanied by resentment and feelings of being 'put upon'.

Fran associated her voice problem as starting following a 'severe throat infection' around the Christmas period. Patients with psychogenic dysphonia frequently report an episode of what they describe as laryngitis as the precipitating factor (Casper and Colton 1990). Fran felt that there had been some recent improvement in the problem but she was anxious to receive reassurance that there was 'nothing seriously wrong'. She reported a history of throat cancer in her family.

Perceptual analysis of Fran's voice quality using the vocal profile analysis (Laver 1980) indicated an overall mild-moderate dysphonia characterised by harshness and whisper (breathiness) with the most significant features being those of creak and voice breaks. The voice did however fluctuate in severity and for short intervals during conversation Fran would exhibit aphonic episodes. The overall pitch of her voice was judged to be mildly lowered with some monotony. Objective assessment of Fran's voice was carried out using electro-laryngography. This is a non-invasive technique that provides information about vocal fold contact during voicing (Fourcin and Abberton 1981) The results of this assessment supported perceptual findings of Fran's voice, revealing a habitual voice frequency of 161 Hz. The average normal value for a female voice is 225 Hz (Boone 1977). Analysis suggested a pattern of vocal fold vibration consistent with excessive muscular skeletal tension. Assessment of Fran's breathing patterns for voice indicated a pattern characteristic of anxiety state. Inspiration for speaking was characterised by excessive upper chest movement and was audible, rapid and 'gasp-like'.

Fran exhibited significant body tension although initially she was largely unaware of this. She made frequent adjustments of body posture and sat predominantly 'on the edge of her seat'. During initial interview she frequently appeared as if she were about to cry. Palpation of her neck, shoulders and larynx indicated moderate muscle tension. Specifically, Fran reported significant discomfort when her larynx was palpated gently by the clinician.

Fran's psychological status was assessed by the speech and language therapist (SLT) using both case history interview and formal questionnaire techniques. The interview questions are typically constructed around areas frequently found to be associated with the onset of psychogenic voice disorder, namely financial difficulties, moving house, bereavement, relationship difficulties, ill-health in oneself or a dependent (House and Andrews 1987; Butcher et al. 1993). The formal questionnaires typically used are the General Health Questionnaire (Goldberg 1981) and Beck's Anxiety Inventory (Beck and Steer 1990). Fran's personal and social history revealed a number of significant stressful life events escalating over the six months preceding her voice difficulties. She was involved in divorce proceedings after the breakdown of her 24-year marriage. She had previously attended 'counselling sessions' with her husband for 'sexual problems in their marriage' but the relationship had ultimately ended with her husband leaving to live with someone else. Fran was currently involved in a new relationship with a married man and expressed concerns over the effect this unstable relationship might be having on her 11-year-old son. Fran felt unsupported by her family over the divorce and had lost close contact with her siblings as a result. She relied on her mother to look after her son on several evenings a week but felt her mother was reluctant to support her in this way. Fran also described a hectic lifestyle working for social services as a carer for the elderly. She reported finding it increasingly difficult to cope with the additional emotional and physical stresses this work placed on her.

Assessment of her psychological status using the General Health Questionnaire-28 (Goldberg 1981) added weight to the impression of high anxiety levels with a total score of 16/56 indicating a degree of psychiatric disturbance. The General Health Questionnaire was designed to focus on 'breaks in normal function rather than lifelong traits' and thus can only be expected to provide useful and meaningful data for a finite group of psychogenic voice patients, namely those with 'psychiatric disturbance' as a transient feature of an otherwise 'healthy functioning'. It does not aim to assess longstanding attributes or how much a patient feels their present state is unlike their usual state. It is thus considered to augment the SLT's psychological interview, drawing the clinician's attention to psychological distress, but offers no replacement for the interview process itself. It has also been observed that it is easier for some patients to communicate the extent of psychological distress through the questionnaire format than through the interview. The application of the GHQ with dysphonic patients is not widely researched. White, Deary and Wilson (1997) identified significant psychiatric symptomatology in

10/18 psychogenic patients using the General Health Questionnaire (GHQ-60) (Goldberg and Williams 1988). Fran's personal and social history therefore indicated an extended period of stress and conflict over speaking out, symptoms commonly found in those patients with psychogenic voice disorder (Butcher et al. 1987).

The voice therapy programme

Following initial ENT examination and more in depth SLT assessment Fran was felt to be an ideal candidate for voice therapy because of her high levels of insight and motivation. An SLT programme of intervention, focusing on the following areas, was agreed with Fran:

- strategies to improve overall voice hydration and care to relieve symptoms of dryness and reduce abusive behaviours such as throat clearing. Fran persisted in smoking throughout her therapy programme but was able to reduce her consumption from 10–15 per day to approximately five per day;
- education regarding the mechanism of voice production, including its sensitivity to negative adjustments in muscle tension;
- further exploration and clarification of the dysfunctional thoughts and behaviours contributing to the anxiety-related symptoms (Butcher et al. 1993);
- reduction of overall muscle tension behaviours using systematic relaxation methods similar to those suggested by Mitchell (1987) and Butcher (1989);
- reduction of muscle tension in the extrinsic and intrinsic laryngeal muscles using laryngeal manipulation techniques (Prater and Swift 1984; Harris and Lieberman 1993) and strategies such as the 'yawn-sigh approach' (Boone 1977).
- teaching breathing techniques for voice to enable control of expiratory airflow for phonation by readjusting the myloaerodynamic mechanism for phonation. Diaphragmatic breathing was also taught as a rapid stress control technique (Butcher 1989).
- utilisation of counselling and stress control techniques (Butcher et al. 1993).

Fran attended five sessions of speech therapy, during which time the above strategies were incorporated very successfully. Counselling techniques were utilised across all sessions as Fran gained more insight into the association between her life stressors and her voice function. On the third session Fran observed that therapy sessions offered her the additional benefit of 'time-out' – an opportunity for her to prioritise herself over and above her other commitments. She began to take a greater interest in her appearance and to assert herself at work and, to a lesser degree, at home.

Having successfully incorporated the voice therapy techniques Fran was exhibiting a significant decrease in tension behaviours overall. Her voice had been 'normal' for three weeks and the sensation of 'a lump' was successfully controlled with the 'yawn-sigh' that Fran used whenever she felt her larynx tighten as a response to emotional pressure. This was frequently associated with the need to 'hold back from crying' that Fran still found difficulty in expressing. Fran had gained a high level of awareness of the psychological factors influencing her voice and was able to control the physical response to these with skill. She had also started to exhibit increased assertiveness skills but it was felt that further psychological input was indicated if Fran was to experience long term relief of her symptoms and if the symptoms were not to be somaticised elsewhere.

Initial interview had identified a number of factors suggesting that Fran's psychogenic voice disorder was typical of the group of patients who suppress their emotions and convert these feelings into musculoskeletal tension. She reported examples of a life crisis, conflict over speaking, burden of responsibility and over-commitment. This had been discussed openly with Fran at her second voice-therapy appointment, where the formal questionnaires she had completed provided a helpful tool for raising some of these issues. A contract of treatment was formalised that clarified two distinct stages of treatment: the first offering symptom relief (namely voice therapy) and the second offering long-term relief of causal factors, namely combined voice and psychological therapy. The patient is typically free to select the type of treatment, knowing the long-term prognosis for each option. They are openly invited to review their decision as voice therapy progresses and their awareness of related issues increases, or they become more able to confront these issues. Referral to psychology for further cognitive-behavioural therapy was therefore discussed with Fran at her second voice therapy appointment but finally agreed with Fran at her fifth appointment.

Psychological assessment and treatment

The psychological interview highlighted an early troubled family life resulting from Fran's father's heavy drinking and violence. In later years he suffered from heart disease and, when this forced him to stop drinking, it was easier to live with him. He had died nine years earlier. Currently, there existed a number of life stresses and relationship difficulties: having separated from her husband, Fran took most of the responsibility for her 11-year-old son, Nicholas; her husband was unreliable with their financial support; she was in a relationship with a married man she knew would not leave his wife; recently, she had fallen out with her brother and sister and her relationship with her mother was particularly difficult.

From early childhood Fran had taken the role of peacemaker. Whenever her father was drunk she felt she had to pacify him in order to protect her mother and to 'stop her getting a thump'. This had been construed by her mother as Fran being on her father's side. Fran complained that her mother often put her down in front of others. However, she had never said anything in response to her mother's criticism. When asked why she never protested or defended herself, she replied: 'Because she's my mum. You should show respect.' Fran's self-description of her positive attributes included being 'a Samaritan' who is 'loyal in family and friendship'. She thought her negative qualities were 'not being able to let go of things' and 'keeping things to myself'. At the end of the assessment, the psychologist provided Fran with a review of his initial findings and a brief description of the cognitive-behavioural model of therapy.

Session one of therapy focused largely on her difficulties as a single, working mother, her son being ill and her estranged husband not showing concern and bothering to visit. At this session she was able to begin exploring her mixed feelings about her father and the difficult relationship she continued to have with her mother, including the indifferent way she felt her mother treated Nicholas and herself. During the session her voice quality deteriorated noticeably when talking about these emotional topics.

Edited transcript of psychological treatment

The transcripts illustrate the central role of counselling in a course of treatment that required the use of very few cognitive-behavioural techniques. It should be noted, however, that she found that observing negative thoughts, looking for positive alternatives and using positive self-instruction (see Butcher et al. 1993 for a description of this emphasis in cognitive-behavioural therapy) was particularly helpful. She commented on this spontaneously at the end of the sixth session when describing her progress. Some individuals require more in the way of cognitive-behavioural therapy skills than this patient but they seem to be a minority and we hope the transcript illustrates that introducing a psychological dimension into treatment is, in general, not too difficult or too fraught with therapeutic hazards. We have chosen only examples of how the sessions focused on the problems in her relationship with her mother because of limited space. However, we could have included very similar and equally striking selections that illustrated how she began voicing her feelings with her estranged husband, her current manfriend and with other acquaintances or friends.

Session 2

Focusing on, and getting details about the central conflict (start of session)

FF A lot of stress over the weekend. I can feel it coming out in my throat.

PB It [the voice] got quite bad last week, didn't it, when we were talking about your mum.

FF My mum? She's good my mum but the trouble is I feel I have to manipulate her into doing something for me rather than doing it freely and openly like I do. If I want her to babysit . . . it's still 'Well, is it still all right for Friday?' . . . I'm never sure with my mum where I am, where I stand.

PB So you mean you have to ask her and double check that it's not just, sort of, accepted?

FF I'm angry because . . . she seems to be there for everyone but not really for . . . [Pausing]

PB For you and Nicholas?

FF Yeah. But if I challenge her on that . . . it's 'Of course . . . I love him' and 'Of course I don't mind' and 'What have you got to ask me for?' . . . I don't know how I stand with my mum . . . I wouldn't say this to her face – I have on occasions and we ended up having a big barney over it – but she's not like how I feel a grandmother should be. She's not . . . [Pausing]

PB How do you think a grandmother should be?

FF Well, like I hope I'm going to be if my son turns round and says 'Mum, can you babysit tomorrow?' I'd say 'Of course I will, I'd love to see the grandchildren . . .'

PB You said last week she's not like a proper grandmother.

FF She's not. I hear all her friends . . . say they've done this with their grandkids, they've done that with their grandkids. I look at me mum [clearing throat] enough to say like, what can I say about you? You know? But if I challenge her on it . . . [clearing throat] You're right, you see, me throat is going. You challenge her in a sort of way then she reverses it and makes me feel guilty.

PB Right. So the challenges don't work very well. They get thrown back at you.

FF No. I don't challenge, mostly . . . But [voice deteriorating, clearing throat] she'll say 'Why are you going off about it, you know I look after him?' [Voice very dysphonic and strained] But I shouldn't keep getting into this situation.

PB Right. So, when you challenge her you say . . . ?

FF Well, basically I say, 'Mum, is it still all right for Friday?' She'll go 'Well . . .'

PB So, she hesitates and ums and ahs.

FF Yes. I think . . . what's the problem? She'll go 'Well, don't you think you should have a night in?' . . . and I go 'All right then, so don't babysit.' 'It's not that I don't want to babysit. I love him being here.' And then she makes me feel she doesn't want him here. So I get very tight.

PB It does illustrate how it, sort of, goes backward and forward – the request for the babysitting – and then her umming and ahing. Then, when you try and question her, she says 'Well, perhaps you shouldn't be going out so much.'

FF That's right. She reverses it to make me feel guilty.

PB So, it's like she's saying you're a bad mother or something.

FF Oh, she's accused me of that but she don't mean it like some people say. She totally thinks I'm wrong about seeing Paul because she knows he's a married man and she says it isn't going to go anywhere. I say I don't want to go anywhere with him. And she says things like 'Mike isn't as bad as this' and I say 'Hang on Mum, last week you wanted to kill him.'

PB So, she's very inconsistent.

FF Very! Extremely, yeah. And that's why I'm very uncomfortable asking her things. I wait to see what kind of mood she's in. Sometimes try a guilt trip on her. I say 'Oh, look Mum I've got something special on this Friday,' and she'll go 'What you making a big fuss for?' And I'll think, well, at least that's over. And then as I drop him off in the morning [before school] I'll go 'All right for tomorrow?' and she'll go 'Tch, I told you it's all right.' and then she could turn like that . . . And I go to work feeling really down . . .

PB What strikes me is you're conveying how anxious she makes you when your trying to do these 'dealings', let's call it, with her and also how you feel always that you can't win, that whatever you do is actually wrong . . . You're wrong if you thought she wouldn't and you're wrong if you think she would . . . You end up tied up in knots when trying to make sense of it.

FF [Talking about her mother criticising what she is wearing] I should be able to turn around and say 'Oh, well, tough. I like what I've got on.' End of. Finish. Walk out the door. That's how I want Nicholas to be.

PB Does she knock the wind out of your sails when she says those things?

FF At times, yeah. Sometimes . . . she'll put me down in front of people . . . I'm the only one in the family that everyone used to come to to sort out the problems but there's no one there to do it for me . . .

PB So, that's been the role you've had hasn't it, where you've been the one who's the peacemaker?

FF Yeah. Ever since I was at school I've been the problem-sorter; even with friends and kids, like, at school.

PB You were suggesting last week that this sort of role of peacemaker was in a way what was going on when your father came home drunk; that you were trying to keep the peace and that was interpreted by your mum as being on his side. Is that right?

FF Yeah.

PB Em. Do you think . . . Were you saying that was what made her jealous of you and your relationship with your father and that's what, sort of, carried on?

FF I think that when my dad died she . . . was very angry . . . because he gave her a very bad time . . .

PB You were also saying that your dad got very close to Nicholas just before he died.

FF Yes, because I was told I couldn't have kids. I was a foster parent . . . Then on the day I lost my two [foster] boys in the high court, I found out I was pregnant after 14 years. Then I nearly lost Nicholas. It all went wrong. I was in hospital for two months. He nearly died. I nearly died. They called my mum and dad and – like my dad was in a wheelchair then – and he made an instant bond because [long pause]. I did love my dad, I love my dad very much and I was the peacemaker and I wouldn't have wanted him to get hurt or her to get hurt. And then I went back to work . . . so they used to look after Nicholas and it used to keep my dad going.

PB Right. So there was a lot of time they had together.

FF Oh yeah. From three months old until he was just over a year . . . So that's the only bit of joy me dad had, looking after Nicholas.

PB And you were suggesting last week that your mum was actually a bit jealous of this?

FF Yes, because when my dad died . . . when we got round there . . . Nicholas came in and he's ran up to her to give her a kiss and she shoved him away . . . I couldn't go round there for a long time 'cause all I kept seeing was my dad there, you know, and she'd be cold and offish toward Nicholas. I suppose in the last couple of years he gave Nicholas all his love . . . so maybe that's why.

PB [Bringing the focus back to her mother's inconsistency] So what do you think she'd say if you said something like 'Mum, look, you're being a bit inconsistent here'?

FF She just rides it off. If you challenge her – which is not that often I do – she just gets out of it. She's like the tide.

PB She's good at twisting things?

FF Yeah. She'll look you straight in the face and say she's been ring-ing you all day, where you been?

PB So she can call black white.

FF Yeah. Oh gawd, can she. Yeah. And you'd think, yeah, maybe she has rung me. But she bloody well hasn't rung you.

PB You start to doubt yourself.

FF Yeah . . . I'd do anything for my mum but I'm under constant pressure if I want to ask her to do something for me . . . She's only got to go 'Mmm' and I'll do it. I wouldn't think twice about it and hesi-tate to do it.

PB So, you're a very loyal daughter.

FF Oh yeah, I am. Extremely.

PB I suppose that must make her behaviour very hard to take really, when she's so difficult and inconsistent?

FF Yeah . . . I'm not as tough as I could be with her. I don't know . . . she's had enough pain, I don't want to cause her any more pain but the thing I'm doing is I'm getting all the hassle . . . So I suppose, yes, there again, I'm being protective.

PB Yeah. It seems to me too that it's . . . the situation making it difficult to say what you think.

FF Yeah, I suppose, yeah, looking at it that way, I've never thought about it. Yeah, I know she's been through a lot my mum.

PB Have you ever told her that?

FF I can't sit down and talk to my mum. Can't have a conversation, like . . . She's snappy . . . She's like a little volcano.

PB So it's even hard to say nice things to her? To say you appreciate she's had a hard time.

FF No, don't get me wrong . . . I'll say I love you . . . and she'll say I love you too.

PB But what about what you were saying before about saying you know she's had a hard time? Have you really talked about that to her?

FF I've tried in the past to talk to her about it but she blocks it off . . . But she wouldn't come to terms with what he used to do . . . I was angry about what my dad had done . . .

PB You were angry about what in particular . . . the way he treated the family?

FF Oh, all that. Yeah, I was angry about all that. I don't know, just the last two years of his life he was the sort of dad I liked because he wasn't allowed to drink or anything, so we'd actually sit and talk and . . . we never had these outbursts of aggression . . . Then when he never made it . . .

PB You finally get the dad you wanted and . . .

FF Yes . . . I finally got a dad that would actually get hold of me and kiss and cuddle me and . . . See, I can't understand why I am so loving when all my closest are so horrible.

PB Have been so cold and rejecting?

FF Yeah, cold, bitter, don't give – excuse my language – a shit about anyone else other than themselves . . . So, I need toughening up. And what I've been trying to do is concentrate on other things . . . So, when I get a downer, I've stripped all my walls now. So when I go home from here I'm going to paint.

PB So you're keeping busy to stop thinking.

FF I'm trying to stop my brain working.

FF [Talking about feeling the need for a break and asking her mother to have Nicholas so she can go out] I get to it I get myself in a state before I get to it. It's Monday and I'm worried about how I'm going to try and get her to have him for this Sunday. And it's not as if she goes out. That's the aggravating thing, you know, she just sits in the house on a Friday, she doesn't do anything.

PB It feels very mean.

FF Yeah . . .

PB And yet you couldn't tell her that?

FF No, 'cause . . . she'd find a way of hurting me . . . a way to say something which would hurt me so deep . . .

PB So, again it's another no-win situation, isn't it?

FF Yeah . . . I've got to look for an opening. The right opening. And that's the way my life is with my mum.

PB So, you're trying all the time to predict where there might be an opening?

FF Yeah.

PB Do you usually predict the response you'll get?

FF Yeah. It's usually always a baddy.

PB Is it. So it's more rare . . .

FF More of a shock if she says 'Oh yeah, no problem.' I go 'Now, are you sure? You really sure?' And when she gives it to me, I go 'Well, you really don't mind? Oh, I really appreciate it. Oh, thanks. Oh, I'm really looking forward to . . . ' and . . .

PB You're overwhelmed with gratitude by the sound of it.

FF Yeah.

PB How does she respond when you're very thankful?

FF [Sharply and quickly] 'Don't know why you make all this fuss. You know I'll have him. You know I love him. You know I don't mind him being here.' That's my mum. Ooh, that's really my mum, then. [Laughing] That's frightening. I really felt that was her then. [More laughter] Bloody hell. Em, yeah, and that's how she'll go. So I can't win either way . . . So, yes, one of my big problems is me mother. [Laughs] I didn't realise it before. I do now.

PB Well, you summed it up very well when you said you can't win because that seems to me to be the sort of knot she ties you in. I think that if there was a way of handling that better, somehow, then it would really help you a lot. And I can see how difficult it is for you to win with her and actually have a relationship that's a lot more rewarding. It seems that there are all these barriers that she puts up to having a good daughter–mother relationship.

FF Yeah, it's a shame because it would be really nice . . . Every Sunday she's over for dinner and every Sunday I don't know what she's going to be like . . . I'm going away Christmas . . . I've made a decision and I'm going. I can't have a Christmas like I had last Christmas . . . Now I've got all the others [siblings] saying 'Whose having Mummy?' I say for once in my life, you sort her out, because I'm not. I thought [laughing] 'Ooh, that's why I booked it and paid for it the same day, because I knew I wouldn't do it otherwise and now it's done.'

PB Are you pleased with that?

FF I am really, I am really pleased. I've done something and I'm not going to worry about her Christmas. She's got two other children. Let them have her.

PB You've carried the responsibility . . .

FF Every Sunday dinner, she's always round, regardless . . .

PB So you've found a way there at least of putting the burden aside . . .

FF I wouldn't let him have a Christmas like last year.

PB So you're putting yourself and Nicholas first.

FF Nicholas first, yeah. I couldn't let him go through a Christmas like that again.

PB No. So do you think you wouldn't have done it for yourself, just if it was for you?

FF If it was just for me I wouldn't have bothered . . .

PB So what do you think that says about you?

FF I'm putting myself back again. It's always someone else first, even if it's Nicholas. I know.

PB Well, it's nice to put your son first but maybe you should be putting yourself equal first.

FF [long, thoughtful pause] Em. I don't know.

PB Is that hard to believe, really?

FF Yeah, yeah, it is. I've never put myself first.

PB Do you think that's another problem you have, in the sense that . . .

FF [Laughing]Will you stop finding all these bloody problems.

PB [Laughing]

FF I was all right . . . I just had a sore throat when I came up to see you. Yeah, I suppose it's a problem. Yeah, I don't never really think of myself first regardless of what situation.

PB Em, well maybe we've touched on the two main problems – if we can talk about you as having problems.

FF [Laughing]

PB One is that you don't put yourself first enough and the other is – as we've been saying – your mum – that she's so difficult . . .

FF Yeah, yeah. I do feel better, I suppose 'cause I'm saying things which have been suppressed and I've not really spoke . . . I couldn't speak to me sister or any of them . . . but, em, I think it's nice to get it out . . . I've just started talking – seems like it wants to come out.

Session 3

Focusing on the common theme of frustration and anger (beginning of session)

FF I'm feeling very angry lately.

PB Are you.

FF Yeah. So, I don't know what you're doing but [laughing] I don't like it. No, I'm very angry toward people at the moment. I'm looking at them differently.

PB Are you. In what sort of way?

FF I'm making them share some of the blame. Instead of it all being on me . . . My mum, I'm angry with. I've tried to be a bit more, you know, positive with her . . . Em, it worked a couple of times but . . . it did affect my throat. You can hear it. It's funny at the moment . . . So I don't seem to be able to win from being not positive to being positive.

PB Right. So . . . you feel disappointed that when you're being positive it doesn't seem to work.

FF Yeah. It's still not working whatever way I seem to go. Now this morning I went to work very tearful and down in the dumps . . .

PB I see. You feel whatever you try doesn't work. When you say you're being positive, can we just explore how you mean that.

FF . . . I never said to her anything about babysitting . . . and she says 'I'll babysit for you. It's no problem' . . . That was on the Sunday. Come the Thursday I thought I'll just see how it is, like I always do, and she went 'Well . . . ' and she started coming out, so I went 'Well, what are you saying now?' So me being positive was me going to her 'What! Are you turning around to me and saying that you can't have him? Now it's a problem, now I've made all the arrangements?'

PB So you spoke up then and said . . .

FF Yeah. Whereas I would have gone 'All right, I'll see what I can do,' or something like that . . . I went, 'Fair enough then, don't look after him' and she walked off.

PB So it sounds like that was very positive, that you were actually challenging her, saying 'Well, you had promised or said it would be alright' and . . . now she's saying something different.

FF That's right. And she went upstairs and then all of a sudden shouted down 'Well, I s'pose it should be all right' and it reverts back on me feeling guilty that I've trapped her into having him.

PB Yeah so . . .

FF So, I didn't win that.

PB I see what you mean. You're trying to be positive but you don't win really.

FF Yeah. I ended up feeling horrible that I trapped her in and maybe she didn't want to have the boy. Maybe it's all too much . . .

PB I was wondering if, perhaps . . . in the past when you tried to speak your mind and say what you thought . . . this is always what happened?

FF It is always what happens.

PB That somehow it seems worse when you do try to communicate things to your mother?

FF Yeah . . . I can physically feel inside that there's got to be a big confrontation . . . that I need to do something and I don't like getting like this . . . I think the reason I push everything down is because there is a part of me that I don't like . . . I will say things and a lot of things have come out.

PB You don't like yourself, did you mean, when you get like this?

FF No. It's very rare that I let my real emotions come out in that respect.

PB But it sounds like quite often you're given cause to get quite angry emotions.

FF Oh yeah, I just suppress them and try and override them . . . If she'd carried on walking I wouldn't have been upset but I would have felt 'Well, that's it, I've said what I want to say.' I wish she'd just walked off.

PB So that would have felt quite good, really.

FF Yeah. I'd have lost out but I wouldn't have felt that I'd manipulated anything . . .

PB With her going up the stairs and doing a turn around.

FF I made her feel guilty for a split second.

PB Right. So you were successful in that way.

FF Yeah . . . I want to come back at them now. I feel – I never used to feel like that – I want to say what's inside me. I want to get rid of it. I don't want to keep it in there any more. I just want to really get it all out.

PB It's nice that you've been, so to speak, 'practising' that and successfully doing that. It sounds as though you want to let go a bit more of the anger, somehow.

FF Yeah, I feel like I want to hit someone. Especially, I want to hit my husband. I think I could enjoy it as well. [Laughing] Mum I've got to deal with another way . . . I just feel . . . I've got to start letting her know what she's doing . . .

PB Is that, perhaps, one of the things that needs to change in you: that you're trying too hard to be too many things to too many people?

FF Well, I've always been like that.

PB Are you saying that you can't change then because you've always been like that?

FF I don't like people doing things for me.

PB Is that why you feel so angry when your mother reluctantly does something to help?

FF Yeah, because I don't really want to . . .

PB Ask in the first place.

FF No.

PB You prefer not to.

FF Yeah.

PB Is it hard to ask for help?

FF Yeah. I suppose it is. Yeah, it is hard. I find it's hard . . .

Session 4

Focusing on her construction of 'being respectful' and the feelings that arise from being assertive (midway through session)

PB I wanted to ask earlier how your mum reacted when you said about Nicholas being upset?

FF . . . She was all right about it.

PB How did that feel for you?

FF It was the thing I wanted to hear her say but I'll go round there after and I'll say, like, 'Are you going to have Nicholas Friday?'

PB So, you're still worrying that she will say . . .

FF Yeah . . . Something will come up and she'll say 'Well . . .'

PB Do you think that with you, perhaps, being a bit different – a bit more direct and getting it off your chest straight away – that, actually, that might have a change?

FF I'm hoping so. I'll know a lot better . . . when I go round there . . . If she says 'Well, you shouldn't be going out,' I'll say, 'All right, I won't go but be it on your head because you're depriving me of one night a week.'

PB So, it sounds as though you're going to let her know in no uncertain terms that you're not happy with how she's treating you.

FF Yeah. I'm going to try and be a bit more positive with my mum and, hopefully, deal with what happens at the time . . .

PB I wonder if there's a different feeling about what is respectful?

FF Yeah, just all of a sudden I've turned round and . . . I don't want to keep feeling how I'm feeling so maybe it's like taking – what's the saying – the bull by the horns? . . . I want to be able to say to her 'Will you do it?' She'll say 'Yes.' Great. End of. And then if she doesn't, if she lets me down [voice deteriorating] then [clearing throat] I want to say 'Hang on a minute, Mum, you . . . well, what am I supposed to do?' You know . . . 'What about me? I've made my arrangements . . . '

PB You put that very well. That's what you really wanted to say. What would you have normally said do you think? Or what did you used to say?

FF Oh, it would have been every day . . . something would have been said . . . like, 'Do you want me to get you a pizza for Friday night?' And she'll probably go 'Well, we'll see', and then that'd make me think, 'What'd she mean, "We'll see"?' . . . [Voice dysphonic, clearing throat.] . . . She controls too much of my life; she really does; verbally, emotionally, my son-wise . . . I do want to be a bit more positive with her and say what I'm feeling, rather than thinking what I should say. That's what I'm aiming for anyway, I mean, I'll just have to face what happens when it happens.

PB Do you feel that you can still be respectful . . . while doing that?

FF I think my mum's got to earn my respect again . . . I don't want to make her suffer . . . but I do want her to start questioning herself.

Session 5

Verbally reinforcing the behavioural change and highlighting the need for consistency (midway through session)

FF I pulled my mum up yesterday. She kept going on in front of her sister. She had a pop at me. I thought, 'No, I'm not having this.' And she went, 'Oh, what was the matter with you yesterday? . . .' I said 'Do you really want to know?' And I looked directly at her. I said 'You blanked me at that funeral,' I said, 'and you were totally out of order.' I said, 'It was hard enough at that funeral,' I said, 'but for you to blank me,' I said, 'that hurt more than anything.' She went, 'Oh, I didn't, I didn't, eh, em,' and all this like, you know, 'I didn't know what I was doing.' I went, 'Just remember, Mum, I've always been the one that stood by you, not them, but you blanked me.'

PB Emm

FF And then she went into her verbal abuse.

PB Yes

FF And I just went 'I'm going to work now.' But she's thought about it because she's all nice and rosy this morning. I went outside . . . and really sobbed . . . but there's part of me that thought 'I'm glad I said it.' And I have been trying to do that more with her . . .

PB So, you're taking charge . . . a bit more . . .

FF A little bit, just a little bit. I mean, I haven't said anything to her about Friday night and I'm just going to take him round there and if she says [anything] I'll go 'Fine, if you don't want to babysit for him, fine. You told me we were back to normal, fine.' And walk away.

PB Well, I'm pleased to hear you are beginning to stand up a bit more for yourself and to say what you think, in particular . . . And it certainly does seem to be getting results.

FF I hope so. I just hope it doesn't all backfire . . .

PB Well, I suppose . . . it's not likely to go wrong if you continue to be consistent with what you're doing because, it seems to me, you've got a good 'formula' there for speaking your mind, saying what you think and, as I said earlier, taking control . . . And the only danger is if you are a bit inconsistent so that your mum starts to think 'Ah, right, she was a bit off at me the other day but I can get away with it because the day after . . . I got my way' or something like that. So . . .

what you have to work out is just being consistent with these things, really.

FF That's what I thought this morning because I was dreading going in there. My old heart was going bang, bang, bang 'Oh, what's going to happen this time?' And I just tried to be casual. I was aware of what I was doing . . . It was on the tip of my tongue to say 'Are you going to have him Friday?' . . . and I thought 'No, I'm just going to turn up Friday with him.'

PB Because that's the old pattern if you go back to saying 'Is it all right?'

FF Yeah, because I didn't this Friday. I nearly did but I didn't.

PB So you're not giving her any ammunition.

FF Not at the moment. I hope not . . .

Session 6

Verbally reinforcing attempts at assertiveness and ability to change (midway through session)

FF . . . I told [Mike] . . . all the things that have angered me. That was Thursday. Dealt with that. On Friday, along comes Mum. 'I hadn't said a word to her all week. No "ifs", no "buts", no little inklings, no drop in. Come Friday morning . . . my aunt's been staying with her . . . And I walked in and . . . just as I was about to depart I thought, 'Right.' I went 'Oh, what treat do you want tonight?' 'What? I can't have him tonight. You're joking.' So, I went 'Well, why?' 'Why? Auntie Sara's staying.' So I said 'Well, so?' So she went 'Well, there's nowhere for him to sleep.' I said, 'He can sleep on the couch.' And she went 'No, I can't have him.' I went 'Right, fine, fair enough, don't have him.' So she said 'What are you going to do then?' I said 'I'm going to have to leave him in the house on his own, aren't I?' 'You can't do that.' I said 'Yeah, I'm going to start thinking about me. Number one.' And I got up and walked off. And she went 'No, no, bring him round here. He can sleep on the couch.' I went 'No, there's no big deal about it,' I said, 'He can stay all by himself.' She went 'You bring him round here!' I went 'All right then,' and went to work.

PB Right. How did you feel about that?

FF Mixed. Bit of triumph and a bit of augh, umm. The most that upset me was that I'd actually used Nicholas.

PB As a lever?

FF Yeah. That hurt. And I am at the moment . . . Well, I was having to do that . . . Monday with Mum – I've got to tell you this because this is also a triumph – on Monday morning I've gone round to my Mum's and for the last few weeks she's been going 'So many days, so many days [to take Nicholas to school before the holidays].' So when me and Nicholas went in Monday, I went . . . as we walked through the door . . . 'Before granny gets a chance to say anything . . . say 'Four more days.' And . . . he laughed and he went 'Oh Mum, you are naughty.' I went 'Well, we'll beat her at it this time.' I thought . . . because that's been hurting me . . . 'I can turn it round.' So she opened the door all miserable – her usual self. [We] went 'Four more days!' 'Oh, shut up!' she's gone. So I went, 'Mum, why are you so happy in the morning?' She went 'Oh, I don't know,' and she went into a moody and that and I just went 'Let's sit in the other room, Nicholas' and thought 'I'm not getting into this.' Anyway, when I came home – I wanted to bring it up to you actually but it's on my answering machine – I won't rub it off – when I got home it's got 'Hello Fran and Nicholas, I do love the pair of you. I know I'm moody' – I can't remember word for word – 'I know I'm moody. I know I'm terrible in the morning. I don't not want to take Nicholas to school. I love taking him to school. I don't mind having him on a Friday. I know I've upset you both. And I do love you both' . . . And I thought 'Ooh, I want everybody to listen to it.' And I haven't rubbed it off yet.

PB Yes, it's quite a thing isn't it?

FF Emm. And coming here today, like, she's had to have the doctor. She's had a chest infection . . . I couldn't hear her shouting she wanted the door shut . . . So I went in and said 'Yes, Mum?' She said 'Fran, you are ignorant. We've been calling you.' When the doctor went out of the door I went back. I went . . . 'Mum, don't embarrass me and say I'm ignorant in front of people. I didn't hear you!' She went 'Oh, I didn't mean it.'

PB Yes. So she's been much more apologetic hasn't she, really, when she has . . .

FF [Interrupting] Well, maybe it's got something to do with me. I mean normally I have just let that go but I'm not a fucking idiot. Sorry, I'm not ignorant. I apologise for swearing as well.

PB [Laughing.]

FF I'm not ignorant. I'm far from it.

PB Coming back to what you said that, perhaps, her being more apologetic has something to do with you. I'm sure that's right.

FF I'd like to think so.

PB Well, that's been the big change, hasn't it, in recent weeks, that you have actually been standing up for yourself and . . . finding that that's actually something that makes things a lot better than before when you did feel it, it . . . wasn't something you could do.

FF Yeah. Gradually things like that are happening . . .

PB You must feel encouraged by that.

FF Yeah, I think I do. Yeah, I'm beginning to, emm. Yeah, I have got some strength in me. [A little later, talking about speaking her mind to a friend] I want to be able to say things and if it doesn't come nice then to be able to apologise but say I mean it.

PB You seem to be finding a good way of saying things to people. As you said earlier . . . if it comes out a bit sharp . . . you'll say you're sorry – that's your view . . . You're saying, 'I'm sorry if that's a bit sharp but that's how I feel' and they can take it or leave it.

FF Well, that's what I did. I ended up saying, 'Well, look Jean, that's my opinion . . . that's my personal opinion . . .' They're going to have to start getting used to . . . I need to be strong like they are. I'm not always going to be a shoulder for everyone . . . People can't keep taking from me . . . I want to be able to say what I want to say. And let bloody someone listen to me for a change.

PB Because that's what you held back on would you say?

FF Yeah. Oh yeah. I wouldn't have said half the things I said to Jean last night.

Session 7

Emphasising the degree of progress and the continued need for consistency (near start of session)

FF [Describing another disagreement with her mother] I said, 'Mum, don't you think that's out of order?', and . . . I just walked away.

PB So again you were incredibly calm and in control of the situation and spoke your mind.

FF Yeah, I walked away because she went verbally at me and I just faced her and I just went, 'Well, sorry, you're out of order,' something like that.

PB So that's also new from what you've told me. You can actually say to your mum 'You're out of order.'

FF I would have stuck up for my mum just to keep the peace.

PB It's important for you to go on in the way you are isn't it?

FF Yeah, because I don't want to keep holding – if I've got feelings there – I don't want to hold them in there. I want to try and let them go . . . Why should I always keep the peace and keep everyone happy because by doing that I'm the one who sits and suffers in silence and I'm beginning to find that . . . What I'm doing is repeating – because if they might not have understood the first little bit maybe the second time I've repeated it, it starts sinking in . . . So it's like, not a game, but it's like a sort of strategy . . .

PB I think the important thing . . . is that you just keep up the consistency . . . in order to remind them . . . this isn't a flash in the pan, you're not going back to your old ways after just trying this out for a few times, because they'll be looking for that to happen.

FF Yeah. I definitely don't want to go back to my old ways . . . I really don't.

Post-treatment assessment

Psychological assessment at follow-up

In total FF received 16 sessions of psychological treatment. As illustrated by the edited transcripts from sessions, she was able to make and maintain, significant cognitive changes in the way she construed her need to carry family responsibilities and be a 'peacemaker'. In addition there were related changes in recognising her tendency to suppress emotions – particularly frustration and anger – and also her need to express these feelings in order to reduce her inner conflicts and its associated voice problems. During the course of treatment she carried out a number of 'behavioural experiments' in assertiveness and in dropping the well-entrenched patterns of not sharing responsibility and being a peacemaker. In doing this she learned to consider her own needs in relationships and to value herself. By session 11 she appeared much less depressed and reported feeling much happier and more in control. At the next appointment, a fortnight later, the change was even more striking and noted by PB as follows: 'Came in looking radiant and sailed into a list of positive things that have happened in the last two weeks, all to do with voicing her feelings and saying what's on her mind.' At the two-month follow-up (session 14) FF had suffered a recent relapse due to a number of unresolved issues with her estranged husband. As she had found no satisfactory way of voicing her feelings, she was once more anxious and agitated and there was a significant deterioration in her voice quality. She was offered further sessions on a fortnightly basis to help her find a way forward with her husband.

By session 16 she again looked relaxed and composed and showed no signs of dysphonia or of having laryngeal discomfort. She reported that after leaving session 15 she had realised she was being 'a mug' when it came to dealing with her husband. That evening she telephoned her husband and told him everything that was on her mind. In particular, she told him that she did not like the way he was treating their son, neither giving him enough attention nor financial support and saying that if he had financial problems then it was up to him to sort them out, not her. She reported that she was able to do this without getting upset and that she felt 'very cool and in control'. As she now felt ready to be discharged, she was offered a review with the speech and language therapist to reassess her vocal function.

Voice assessment at follow-up

Fran was reviewed by the speech and language therapist approximately three months after discharge from her psychology appointments. She reported a continuing pattern of life stresses that, if anything, had escalated since the cessation of psychological treatment. However, her personal outlook and attitude towards these stressors had strikingly changed since the start of treatment. As she described the life-events of the past few months, she talked with confidence about how she had used assertiveness skills, as well as other coping strategies. For example:

FF [Talking about mother] She behaves a lot better because I don't let her use me and I don't let her wind me up so much . . . There are still times when she beats me but she doesn't hurt me so much. I'm grateful to PB because I didn't realise it was such a problem and it was . . . , it really was.

Fran also reported a continuing heightened awareness of her body's physiological responses to stress and an increased ability to recognise these early and respond appropriately. For example:

FF [Talking about her occasional dysphonia and overall communication] The only time I'm aware of it is . . . when there is a problem. Then I think . . . 'I wonder' . . . as soon as it starts causing me a problem, I don't let it go on and on. I take my time, sit with it and deal with it.

LC So you control it.

FF I'm calming it down, trying to talk slower . . . I don't know . . . people are beginning to listen better.

Whilst describing these occasional episodes of fluctuating voice difficulty, Fran's habitual voice quality was much improved and fell within normal limits in all parameters. Reassessment with the Vocal Profile Assessment indicated only mild features of creaky phonation at the end of phrases, use of abdomino-diaphragmatic breathing and a slower, more relaxed rate of speech. Objective reassessment using the electrolaryngograph indicated an increased habitual pitch of 207 Hz, a rise of 46 Hz, despite no direct work on pitch. This can be explained by her improved breath control, laryngeal relaxation and improved psychological status. In addition, Fran's overall body posture was relaxed with an absence of any throat discomfort.

Finally, Fran repeated the General Health Questionnaire, with a total score of zero using the standard GHQ scoring system, and thus falling well within the normal range. This supported her reports of psychological improvement at interview

Conclusions

The case study illustrates how using a combination of voice and psychological therapies can be an effective therapeutic approach in the management of the client with a diagnosis of psychogenic dysphonia. It also suggests that once patients recognise the causes underlying their voice difficulties and acquire various skills to deal with these causes, and/or to alter cognitive-behavioural patterns which maintain their problem, they can sustain their progress even when external pressures continue or worsen. We believe that a more 'one dimensional' or less comprehensive treatment approach would be less successful and less self-protective for the patient. Much of this is summed up by Fran at her final interview with LC when she said:

FF He [PB] helped me control the stress . . . my anger. I'm not afraid to say what I feel. When I do get to that stage and am losing it a bit, then I come back to your methods and do all my exercises. I couldn't have done it without you both.

Chapter 4
Chris, Usha and Bridget: supporting bullied students

SONIA SHARP

Introduction – bullying is a wide spread problem in schools – bullying behaviour takes many forms – bullying has negative effects – providing a framework for action – general principles for supporting bullied students – teaching assertiveness – boosting self esteem – adapting the approaches to meet the student's individual needs – evaluation of assertiveness work with bullied students – summary.

Introduction

I developed an interest in language whilst studying for my A-levels in modern foreign languages. I wished to continue to work with languages at university but wanted to extend my studies beyond the traditional literature and language courses being offered. Whilst investigating possible options I discovered a course at Aston University in Birmingham entitled 'psychology of human communications'. This course could be studied jointly with linguistics and seemed ideal. I was not disappointed with the course I had chosen. I discovered the fascinating world of psychology and developed a particular interest in the educational progress of children and young people. With a view to training as an educational psychologist I attended Worcester College of Higher Education where I trained for a post-graduate certificate of education in English and drama. Teaching experience is one of the requirements for the qualification in educational psychology.

My first post was as a general teacher in an independent school for children with speech and language difficulties. During this year I worked closely with speech therapists in the school to develop learning programmes that would meet the students' educational and language needs. Although the quality of teaching and therapy within the school was exceptional, I was disturbed by the seeming paradox of placing children with language and communication difficulties in a context where they were segregated from peers who could act as appropriate models for language use. My next posts were in mainstream comprehensive schools in Leeds and Barnsley.

Having taught for four years, I began training as an educational psychologist at Sheffield University. It was during this time that I began to be interested in student stress and bullying. In 1991, I began work as principal research fellow on the DFE Sheffield anti-bullying project, directed by Peter Smith in the Department of Psychology at Sheffield University. The project ran for two-and-a-half years and involved me in working closely with 24 schools to develop and evaluate effective anti-bullying strategies. After the project I returned to my post as educational psychologist in Barnsley. Since then I have worked as senior educational psychologist in Lincolnshire and have recently been appointed chief educational psychologist in Buckinghamshire. I have continued to research in the area of bullying, have written widely on the subject and have lectured nationally and internationally. Throughout my work as an educational psychologist I have remained committed to working collaboratively with schools to establish organisational and curriculum approaches to building constructive peer relationships and including students who experience special educational needs.

Bullying is a widespread problem in schools

Many students are bullied in school and students with speech and communication difficulties are no exception. Research into bullying experiences of students with special educational needs have suggested that they are more at risk of being bullied. In a study of 179 students, Nabuzoka and Smith found that students who experienced learning difficulties reported higher levels of bullying than those without. They also noted that these students tended to be less popular and more rejected by peers. Whitney et al. (1994) also investigated bullying experiences of children identified as experiencing special educational needs. In this study 186 students, in pairs matched for age, gender and ethnic group, were interviewed before and after their school had carried out some anti-bullying work. Ninety-three of the students had special educational needs and 93 did not. Whitney and her colleagues found that students with special educational needs were significantly more likely to be bullied than children without special educational needs, especially within the secondary school setting. Many of these students were bullied persistently – several times a week throughout the school term. None of the students within this study was specifically identified as experiencing difficulties with speech and language, although their teachers did comment on their poor social skills.

As many as one-in-four primary-aged students and one-in-ten secondary-aged students report that they have been bullied more than once or twice during each school term (Whitney and Smith 1993). Between four and six per cent report being bullied more frequently – at least several times a week. These students are not only bullied in school but on the way to and from school as well. A similar number of secondary-aged students report that the bullying lasts for more than a year (Thompson 1995).

Bullying behaviour takes many different forms

Bullying can include many different types of aggressive anti-social behaviours. Common forms of bullying include name-calling, other verbal 'put downs', deliberate physical attack, threats, damage to possessions, social exclusion, rumour spreading and extortion. Bullying is distinguished from other types of aggressive behaviour as involving a systematic abuse of power, being intentional and occurring over a fairly long period of time. Bullying often involves the same people doing similar things to someone over and over again. Unfortunately, once a student has begun to be bullied by one group of peers they can become ostracised or picked on by others in their class or year group. This 'social dynamic' of bullying means that once the bullying relationship is established it can be very resistant to change.

Bullying has negative effects

Nobody enjoys being bullied. It is a fairly unpleasant experience. In a survey of 723 students, Sharp (1995) found that 34 per cent of students had been bullied and had found this experience stressful. Common reactions to bullying were to feel irritable, panicky or nervous; to have recurrent memories of the bullying and to find it difficult to concentrate in school. Twenty-two per cent of students reported that they actually felt ill after being bullied. Bullying was identified as a chronic stressor leading to negative stress effects for many students. Olweus (1980) found that students who were persistently bullied were more anxious and insecure than other students, had a negative view of themselves, were often lonely and neglected by peers and generally had low self-esteem. Rigby and Slee (1991) reported that bullied students showed slightly lower self esteem than non-bullied peers but also noted that gender was more associated with variations in self esteem than victimisation. In a further study (Rigby and Slee 1993) found that students who were being bullied 'at least once a week' reported higher levels of somatic complaints, general depression and suicidal thoughts than non-bullied peers. Haselager and Yan Lieshout (1992) found that bullied students are more likely to show signs of depressive distress, negative self evaluations and physical complaints than other classmates. They were also more likely to be rejected by peers, to be shy and withdrawn and less likely to be chosen as a best friend.

Neary and Joseph (1994) investigated self worth, depression and victimisation in 60 11- and-12-year-old girls. They found that the girls who had scored more highly on a victimisation scale also reported lower global self worth, poorer perceptions of themselves in relation to academic competence, social relationships, attractiveness and conduct. Bullying can affect student happiness, self esteem and well being.

Reid (1989) investigated reasons for truancy and found that 15% of persistent absentees said they had stayed away from school initially because of being bullied; 19 per cent continued to stay away from school because of this. Balding et al. (1996) carried out a questionnaire survey of 11 11 to 16 year olds from 65 schools. Some of the questions in the survey related to fear of going to school, fear of being bullied and self-esteem. They found that of 4989 Year 8 students, 21.3 per cent of boys and 28.2 per cent of girls reported that they were sometimes afraid to go to school because of bullying. For 2.4 per cent of boys and 3.1 per cent of girls they felt this 'very often'. These students reported higher frequencies of illness and disease and generally presented as more anxious. Pervin and Turner (1994) surveyed 107 13- and 14-year-old students in one secondary school. Seventy-seven per cent of the boys and 89 per cent of the girls who had experienced bullying found it either worrying or frightening. Two students had changed schools because of the bullying.

All of these studies demonstrate that bullying is a problem that we should all take seriously. Even though an incident may seem minor or trivial to those not directly involved, bullying can cause great distress and can prevent students from meeting their full educational potential. Fortunately, there have been a number of studies that suggest that schools and families can take action against bullying and the remainder of this chapter will explore some of these.

Providing a framework for action

All of the intervention studies that have been carried out have emphasised the need for a whole school approach to preventing and responding to bullying. It seems that a key factor in reducing levels of bullying is engaging students, staff and parents in discussions about the problem and what can be done about it. In the anti-bullying project carried out in Sheffield (Smith and Sharp 1994), schools that had actively involved all students and staff and as many parents as possible in awareness raising and consultation activities experienced the largest reductions in levels of bullying. As an outcome of these activities, staff, students and parents developed a shared understanding of bullying behaviour and were able to establish a comprehensive set of guidelines for action that clarified what people should do to prevent and respond to bullying. Strategies for supporting bullied students were included in these guidelines for action and the remainder of this chapter will focus on these. However, it is important to emphasise that interventions that aim to support bullied students may not stop the bullying although they may help the bullied student to feel more confident and competent when faced with bullying behaviour. Effective intervention requires work with everyone who is involved in the bullying situation, including the bystanders.

General principles for supporting bullied students

Supporting bullied students requires a balance between enabling them to cope with being bullied themselves and joining with them so they do not have to do it by themselves. Students who are bullied persistently may already have low self-esteem and self-confidence. If they have to rely totally on others for action against bullying they can be left feeling helpless and incompetent, which may reduce their self-esteem further. However, bullying behaviour by nature is very difficult for an individual student acting alone to stop. A group response to bullying will be more effective. In working with bullied students it is important to emphasise that the idea that an individual can 'stand up to bullying' is unrealistic. There are strategies the individual student can use to cope more effectively and to manage the situation but these on their own will not necessarily stop the bullying.

Teaching students to be assertive in their relationships can help them to feel more confident in themselves and provide the skills to de-escalate bullying situations. Assertiveness is a set of techniques based on a specific philosophy of human rights. These techniques build on a standard formula and provide an individual with a clearly defined structure to use in different social contexts. They therefore provide the user with a 'script' that they can fit to meet their personal needs. For bullied students these scripts provide a sense of security that leaves students feeling more control and power and less anger or despair. For students with speech and communication difficulties, the opportunities to rehearse what to say and how to say it can increase their confidence in responding to bullying. As assertiveness training includes work on non-verbal behaviour as well as verbal behaviour it can be an empowering experience for students with even the most profound expressive problems.

In responding assertively, the student will stand up for his/her rights without violating the rights of the other student. By definition, bullying behaviour involves an abuse of power whereby one person or group of people dominates another. By responding to the other student as an equal the bullied student is able to redress the imbalance of power associated with bullying incidents. The assertive student will respond to the bullying student by stating their intentions, wishes and/or feelings clearly and directly. They remain resistant to manipulative or aggressive tactics. Assertive responses not only rely on verbal messages but on eye contact and body language as well. Students can be taught to:

- make assertive statements;
- resist manipulation and threats;
- respond to name calling;
- leave a bullying situation;
- enlist support from bystanders;
- boost their own self-esteem;
- remain calm in stressful situations.

The individual student has to judge the bullying situation him/herself and decide what is the best response. Sometimes this may be to run away as quickly as possible and seek assistance from an adult. By teaching students assertive behaviour we simply broaden their repertoire of possible responses to a given situation.

Students can be taught to apply four principles to any bullying incident. These four principles are:

- assess the situation;
- respond assertively;
- enlist support (either immediately or soon after);
- leave the situation as quickly as possible.

Assertive behaviour can be introduced to all students through the main curriculum. This approach involves the teacher demonstrating a technique to the whole class, enabling the students to practise it in pairs or threes and then discussing with students, either as a whole class group or in smaller groups, how effective the technique might be, what variations might be possible, when it would be most appropriate for the technique to be used and so forth.

Some teachers or therapists may wish to set up a smaller group setting that brings together a number of students who have experienced persistent bullying. This kind of group can be very supportive, providing a safe forum for individual students to talk about their experiences and develop and rehearse ways of dealing with bullying. It allows the adult more time to help each student to shape the techniques to fit their own personal circumstances and abilities whilst still providing the students with opportunities to practise the techniques through role-play.

When setting up this kind of group both teachers and therapists will need to consider carefully who will be involved. The ideal number of students is between six and eight. Students of all ages can benefit from this kind of group. There is no reason why different aged students cannot be involved in the same group, although it is easier to work with students of a similar level of language development and maturity. The group will probably need to meet at least five or six times because, in the earlier meetings, students need time to get to know each other. If a group is made up of children from different schools, then the period of group formation will need very careful management. Some students may respond to the new group situation with aggressive or disruptive behaviour.

The length of meeting depends upon the maturity and attention span of the students involved and the amount of time available. Valuable gains can be made through a series of 20-minute sessions.

Finally, both teachers and therapists can teach individual students how to behave more assertively. This will involve the adult finding time to meet with the student (and possibly a friend) to discuss the bullying being experienced and to introduce them to appropriate assertive behaviours. In this kind of one-to-one situation, the adult will need to reverse roles with the student to demonstrate the technique and then role-play the bullying student to allow the bullied student to practise the technique.

Assessing the need for assertiveness work and how best to introduce it will involve discussion with the people who know the student well, such as teachers and family members and the students themselves. The kinds of concerns that may be expressed may include social isolation, other difficulties in managing social relationships, experiences of being bullied fairly persistently, being 'easily led' by peers. Assertiveness work is only effective if the student is willing to be involved, so part of the assessment will be to ascertain his or her views on involvement. Detail about the types of social experiences that are causing concern as well as those that are successful can aid planning of the types of strategies and approaches that can be included in the intervention. It is often worth exploring with the school whether or not there are other students who experience similar difficulties, because assertiveness training in small groups has many benefits. First, it enables practice with peers and, secondly, the group itself can become a supportive arena for relationship development.

Teaching assertiveness

The most effective method for teaching students assertive behaviour is based on maximising the opportunities for modelling and practice within the group setting. The students need to feel familiar with the 'script' they are being taught to enhance their confidence in using it. First, the student needs to observe or model the assertive behaviour. This might involve the teacher or therapist demonstrating it. Next, she or he needs several opportunities to practise and adapt the behaviour. Practice should include imagining using the assertive behaviour in different settings. Some form of feedback should be offered to the student to help them refine their approach. Attention should be paid to body language and eye contact as well as verbal messages. Finally, she or he should be encouraged to discuss how this type of assertive behaviour could be used, including when it would not be appropriate. A combination of rehearsal based on real-life experiences and discussion of when and how the students will put the assertive behaviour into practice might assist with the generalisation process.

Body language and eye contact

All of the assertive behaviours described in the next section depend on a combination of verbal message and confident body language. When responding assertively to a situation, students should stand upright and look the other person in the eye. The student's facial expression should be neutral, smiling only if appropriate. Hands and arms should be relaxed and by the side or in pockets. Crossed arms, covering the mouth with a hand or fidgeting are defensive behaviours. Hands on hips or pointing can be perceived as aggressive.

Assertive statements

Making an assertive statement involves being clear, honest and direct. It involves stating quite specifically and calmly what you want or how you feel about an event or situation. For example, a student might be being disturbed by another student who is talking noisily while he or she wants to work. An assertive response would be, 'I would like you to be quiet', an aggressive response would be 'shut up or I'll hit you', a passive response would be to suffer in silence or to move. For bullied students, assertive statements can be helpful when responding to name calling, teasing or mild physical provocation. Students can learn to say, 'I don't like it when you do that. I want you to stop.'

Resisting manipulation and threats

When children are under pressure they can choose between two assertive techniques. The first is to say 'no' or even 'no, I don't want to'; the second is slightly more sophisticated and is based upon the repetition of an assertive statement.

Learning to say 'no' can be harder than it sounds. Children, especially girls, are often encouraged to be 'kind' and 'unselfish'. Unfortunately, this can sometimes lead to children doing things against their wishes or best interests. To be able to say 'no', children have to learn that they have the right to say 'no' and also when to use that right. If they feel comfortable complying with another person's request, then they should say 'yes'. They also may be able to identify a compromise solution that will keep everybody happy. If, however, they have that sinking feeling of 'oh, no, I really don't want to do this' then they should say 'no'.

Manipulation, threat and persuasion are often based on moral or emotional reasoning. Students may face a barrage of threats and promises. One way of resisting is to keep repeating the same assertive statement until the other children give up asking. This technique is called 'broken record' because it is reminiscent of a record being stuck. Here is an example of 'broken record' in practice.

Rachel:	Give us that chocolate!
Jo:	I don't give other people my chocolate.
Rachel:	Go on, don't be such a spoilsport!
Jo:	I don't give other people my chocolate.
Rachel:	But I shared mine with you the other day.
Jo:	I don't give other people my chocolate.
Rachel:	I won't let you come to my party!
Jo:	I want to come to your party but I don't give other people my chocolate.
Rachel:	(Walks off)

The broken record here, was 'I don't give other people my chocolate'. Threats and manipulation may be accompanied by aggressive posture and expression. Teach the students to maintain confident body language, even if the bullying student comes very close or gives nasty looks. Usually, the other student will stop pressuring the child using the broken record after three attempts. Nevertheless, children who are being taught this kind of technique against bullying also need to assess when is the best time to walk away from the situation. They should practise the technique and walking away!

Responding to name calling

If assertively telling the other person to stop name calling does not work, then a technique called 'fogging' can be helpful. When fogging, the bullied student responds to each taunt or name with a neutral statement that aims to de-escalate the situation rather than escalate it. Statements such as 'you might think so'; 'possibly'; 'it might look that way to you'; 'so?' are fogging type statements. The tormentor soon becomes fatigued if the bullied student remains calm and nonchalant in the face of their abuse.

In situations where it is difficult to make a verbal response students can be taught to 'positive self talk' – just as it sounds, this involves saying nice things to yourself! By concentrating mentally on positive messages such as 'I can stay calm', or 'I am wonderful' it is possible to block out external messages to a certain extent and to feel more confident.

Enlisting support

Emphasise that individual responses to bullying are far less effective than group responses to bullying. There may be other students or adults who are nearby during a bullying incident. Shouting to attract their attention can quickly put an end to the incident and provide backup for assertive behaviour. Statements such as 'Look what they're doing! It's not fair, is it?' can mobilise bystanders into activity and create an instant challenge to the bullying behaviour. Approaching peers who, whilst not involved directly, can often be bystanders, can lead to increased bystander support in the future.

Walking away

This is best done quickly and calmly. Students need to practise when and how to walk away. Teach the students to walk confidently and unhesitatingly. If possible, choose an exit to the side rather than backing off or pushing past the bullying students. There may be times when the most prudent action is to run away as fast as possible. Discuss with the students how they should choose which course of action to take.

Unfortunately, bullied students may find themselves in situations where they are being physically threatened. Local community police officers or women's self defence groups may offer training on safe techniques for resisting physical violence.

Boosting self-esteem

Students who experience persistent bullying often have low self-esteem. Activities that involve giving and receiving compliments; positive self-statements; circle activities where each student completes a sentence such as 'I like myself because I . . .' help to remind the students that they are valued human beings.

Teaching students how to relax helps them to stay calm, and therefore appear confident, in bullying situations. There are many strategies available for stress management and relaxation. They usually fall into three categories:

- breathing control;
- physical relaxation;
- visualisation.

Teaching students to control their breathing involves counting slowly while the student breathes in and out. A count of three to breathe in and four to breathe out can slow the heartbeat and encourage relaxation.

Physical relaxation can be introduced through tensing and then relaxing different parts of the body. Students need to learn how to feel the difference between a tense muscle and a relaxed one. Holding the hand tight and then letting it go floppy can be a simple introduction to relaxation. This can be progressively extended to the rest of the body. Working with students so that they learn which parts of their body are particularly tense can be helpful in focusing relaxation. Common 'tense points' include the jaw, shoulders and stomach.

Visualisation involves using mental images to aid relaxation. Ask the student to visualise a place where he or she feels comfortable, safe and calm. Encourage the student to pay attention to shapes, colours, sounds, smells, textures in the place so they really have a clear image of the place in their mind. By remembering how safe and comfortable they feel in that place they can induce similar feelings of calm and safety again. When they are feeling anxious, by calling up the image of the place and the feelings of relaxation and comfort that go with it, they can help themselves to relax.

Adapting the approaches to meet the student's individual needs

Every student is different and the bullying situations they face will vary. When working with the student to develop assertive behaviour and other strategies for coping with bullying you will often need to adapt the approaches or include additional work on social skills to suit their individual situations. Here are some examples of work with individual students that illustrate this:

- Chris is a 14-year-old secondary-school student. He had no specific speech and communication difficulty but he would only whisper. He had been constantly taunted and picked on by many students in his year group throughout his school days. His teachers reported that he had no friends, preferring to spend lunchtimes by himself. Chris himself did not show much distress when bullied but his family and teachers were all concerned and wanted him to be involved in a school-based group for managing bullying. Chris was neutral about attending but did come along and participated in all activities. As well as teaching him assertive strategies for handling this taunting, we also concentrated on breathing and voice projection work. Once we had worked on projecting a louder voice we introduced the assertive strategies. Each verbal response was practised first in a whisper and then in a louder voice. Although we were never able to encourage Chris to shout, he did begin to speak in a louder voice.

- Usha is an eight-year-old primary-school student. She has a word-finding difficulty and was teased because she paused a lot in her conversation, lost track of her utterances and would use the wrong word to express herself. We worked intensively on building self-esteem, stress management and positive self-talk for times when her peers would laugh at her mistakes. We also practised ways of explaining that she did not like it when peers laughed at her difficulties with language and asking them not to laugh at her. The class teacher held a series of class discussions about bullying and teasing during which several students talked about their experiences of bullying and how this had hurt them. During these discussions Usha was able to explain to her classmates why she had difficulty expressing herself and how embarrassed she was when people laughed at her and teased her. Even up to a year later Usha reported that the strategies were helpful: she was teased less by the class and some students had even stood up for her in the playground. Her family reported that she was much happier about coming to school and seemed to have more friends.

- Bridget is a 15-year-old student with semantic-pragmatic difficulties. She was ostracised from her peer group because she often used contextually inappropriate utterances and her peers regarded her as 'odd'. The bullying had started when she transferred from primary school to secondary school. On transfer she lost contact with her classmates and this was a particular blow because she had progressed through nursery, infant and junior school with the same peer group. She had been accepted and included as a member of the school community. Because of her success in junior school, her teachers had not seen it necessary to support her in developing relationships in the secondary phase. Although there were other children from her primary class who transferred to the secondary school with her, they had been placed in other forms. From the outset of her secondary career Bridget had been ostracised and rejected by her new peers. This became a pattern and by the time I worked with Bridget she had spent four years of education being bullied. During my work with Bridget her form tutor worked with the whole tutor group on a topic looking at prejudice against disability and bullying, during which the way students behaved towards Bridget was discussed and strategies for including her socially within the group were agreed. Work on sustaining conversation and turn taking was included in the assertiveness work with Bridget. Her teachers were asked to support this in the classroom setting by including opportunities for conversation and discussion and guiding Bridget where necessary. Two students were appointed as buddies for Bridget – they not only tried to involve her in social activities but were also taught how to model and reinforce socially appropriate conversation. We evaluated the effectiveness of this work by interviewing Bridget, the students in the class and her teachers. The outcomes were seen as positive with Bridget demonstrating an increase in appropriate utterances, greater involvement in both structured and unstructured activities, less bullying and an increase in self esteem for Bridget.

Evaluation of assertiveness work with bullied students

During the DFE-funded Sheffield anti-bullying project, the assertiveness training work was evaluated by using a combination of interviews, self esteem measures, teacher comments and student responses to hypothetical situations (Tonge 1992; Childs 1993; Whitney et al. 1994). Nineteen students were followed up from six different schools, aged between seven and 16 years. Teachers noted a visible increase of confidence in the students with greater student participation in classroom and social activities. The outcomes for students with special educational needs were particularly positive. The majority of the students said they felt more confident and this was supported by a significant increase in self esteem. Julie (aged 15) commented:

> I don't hardly talk in the first year or second year and that's why they picked on me . . . [since the assertiveness work] I've started talking a lot and making new friends.

John (aged 14) described why he felt his relationship with someone who had been bullying him had changed:

I showed him that I weren't afraid of him. 'Cos he used to work on my fear . . . but if it happened again, I mean, it's not as if I'm small anymore and I can't do anything . . . I feel confident and I can stop them if they start on me.

Eighty-five per cent of the students interviewed said that they used the assertive strategies and that this had not only helped them to feel better but also had reduced the bullying they experienced. Chris (aged 14) said:

it taught me what to really do when you've got a difficult situation . . . I've only needed to use it once . . . when telling them . . . keep using the same statement over and over again . . . well, they were just asking me if they could borrow some money and I knew they wouldn't give it me back, so, I just said 'no'.

Michael, aged 14 years, reflected:

it gets you out of bullying at break and you use words that you didn't know you could use before . . . ever since I've been using those words, yeah, I haven't been bullied for a long time . . . I feel a bit bigger, instead of feeling little . . . I feel as though I can look at them from a great height instead of them standing on the ladder and looking down at me.

Summary

Bullying is an unpleasant experience and students with special educational needs are more likely to be bullied than their peers. If unchallenged, bullying leads to lower self esteem, reduced educational progress and stress. To prevent bullying happening and to stop it once it has begun, requires a co-ordinated approach within the school. In conjunction with these 'whole school' approaches we can support persistently bullied students by teaching them to manage the bullying situation assertively. This may or may not help to stop the bullying re-occurring, however it will assist the student to feel more confident and competent so that the impact of the bullying behaviour is reduced and the bullying situation is de-escalated.

Chapter 5
Harry's story: becoming a counsellor following a stroke

HARRY CLARKE

Harry before the stroke – the stroke – early days in counselling training – a person-centred philosophy – reliving the stroke: a Gestalt exercise – starting work at City Dysphasic Group (CDG) – disability – difficulties – the counselling process – supervision – spirituality – today and tomorrow.

Harry before the stroke

Having worked in the music business and as an exhibition manager I'd been familiar with a certain amount of risk taking. I had looked at success from a purely monetary aspect. I had also enjoyed the 'high profile' aspect of my work, indeed the uncertainty and risk was a large part of the appeal and, consequently, there were as many great highs as there were lows. At the beginning of my fateful 35th year I began to question my life's direction. I felt uneasy. Things in my working life were changing and I was becoming more and more disenchanted with my views as to what the future held. Both my parents had died within the last five years and at 35 I realised I was roughly in the middle of my life. I was beginning to feel lost. On reflection I was sliding into depression without really knowing it. I later coined the analogy of being in a small boat in the middle of the Pacific Ocean and having lost both sail and oars and with a broken rudder this tiny craft was drifting aimlessly, just bobbing direction-less. I seemed to be willing something to happen. Anything. My internal view of the world was coming from a position of pain that coloured my external view, the one perpetuated by the other. This would have been a good time to seek the assistance of a counsellor had I known what counselling was about. I'd heard the term 'counselling' perhaps for the first time after the King's Cross fire and had linked it to being something victims of trauma were offered to help them come to terms with tragic events they'd been involved in, certainly nothing that I could see being of help to me. And so this lost feeling continued until the morning of Friday, 27 June 1988.

The stroke

I opened my eyes and knew there was something dreadfully wrong. In that hazy limbo between sleep and wakefulness, it felt as though I was still in some restless disturbed dream and that if I were to go back to sleep completely, I would wake later and it would be all gone. I don't know how long it was but eventually the call of nature forced me into waking. That awful 'wrong feeling' was still there. Dragging myself up – I wondered why it was such a struggle – it felt as if I'd slept heavily on my right arm. I couldn't feel it at all and couldn't seem to get the circulation going. I tried to stand but immediately fell heavily, hurting myself. I was now frightened and confused but managed to stay calm. I pulled myself up and tried to stand up once more. I fell, hard and painfully. I tried several more times until at last I could stand no more. I had no conception whatsoever of what was happening to me but my mind was alert and sharply focused. It was clear that I needed help, so I half crawled, half dragged myself to the telephone and with my left hand, dialled the number of a friend. He picked up the phone and I opened my mouth expecting to hear the words, 'Chris, there is something wrong with me, can you help?' Instead, to my horror, all I heard was a garbled mumbling, unintelligible nonsense. Now I panicked. The physical problem was a puzzle but this sudden inability to communicate something that was so crystal clear in my mind filled me with terror. I wrestled with my mouth, desperately trying to say what I meant, but there was nothing but this grotesque, Neanderthal garbage. Mercifully, Chris guessed who it was. He had the presence of mind to tell me he would call an ambulance and told me to get to the front door. This I did, with difficulty, and I slumped there and just waited in silence, trying to grasp what on earth was happening to me.

I vividly remember everything in the flat being as it always had been. Safe, normal and in order, exactly as it should be, and me in this hideous nightmarish, closed world. The ambulance arrived and very quickly I was on my way to Westminster Hospital. Those first hours in hospital are now a blur. What seemed like endless hours of examination by doctors, who talked amongst themselves but not to me. Hours of wondering what on earth was happening to me. My mind was screaming out loud but my mouth was a pathetic jumble.

The weekend came and went. When I would normally be out enjoying myself with friends, I lay still in that hospital ward drifting in and out of sleep, a restless fitful sleep, all the time not knowing what was going on. When I tried to communicate with my visitors, their faces were a mirror of my own puzzlement and confusion. On the following Friday a doctor came to see me with the results of the scan. He sat down and explained carefully that I had suffered a major cerebrovascular accident. This meant nothing to me, but then he said it meant a stroke. I asked why it had happened. He said there was no specific reason and when I asked when I could leave the hospital, when I could walk, talk and use my arm and leg again, all he said was that he couldn't say. These were blunt and truthful answers but they only served to deepen my frustration. He said that the one thing he could say was that I would be in hospital for a long time. I scoffed at the suggestion and told him I would be out in a couple of weeks. A fortnight later, I was forced to reassess the situation. It was plain to see that I had a long and hard struggle ahead of me but from the first diagnosis I was determined to beat these awful disabilities and if my predictions of how long it would take were a little hasty, it didn't lessen my determination to get better. I just accepted that it would take a little longer.

In those early days, my first goal was to get up and walk. That independence seemed of paramount importance, but gradually the inability to communicate coherently became increasingly frustrating. Although my speech was improving, progress was so slow. I soon realised that this facet of my recovery was by far the most important.

I have memories of that eventful year and looking back can document significant moments that led me to the path I am now on. I would like to mention a few key incidents that I believe have shaped my direction. Three weeks after the stroke and feeling particularly distressed as realisation finally set in of the enormity of my illness, I was wheeled into my regular speech therapy session where it was felt most headway was being made. The speech therapist had arranged her desk, as usual, with a few instruments needed for the next hour's work. I knew the procedure, but somewhere deep inside a small voice was screaming 'What about me?' In anger I pushed everything off her desk and shook my head, trying to express a need I would have had trouble conveying even if I had no speech problems. I was crying out for counselling but there was no one there. My speech therapist tried as best she could by at least being there for me and listened as I poured out in broken words, my confused and distressed feelings. At least for that one hour I had made someone aware of how I was really feeling and it felt good. Why on earth they never recognised this need I'll never know. I remember thinking 'Yes, speech therapy, physiotherapy and occupational therapy are a tremendous help but I know there's something else – another therapy which I'm sure they'll be introducing soon.' It never came.

It's easy now to see what that missing therapy was, but it has to be remembered this was my first experience of hospital and so much had been and was happening. I totally relied on the hospital staff to do what was best for me and never questioned their expertise and knowledge. They obviously knew what I needed, and they did, but purely on a physical level.

After three months I left hospital and moved into the Wolfson Rehabilitation Centre in Wimbledon. I had heard great things about this place and felt this was where I'd make my big recovery. I'd made great inroads at Westminster, especially my speech, so much so that at my initial assessment it was decided I no longer needed speech therapy and was told I would regain my speech almost completely. This was great news on its own, but it also meant I could concentrate more of my efforts on walking and regaining the use of my right arm and hand.

The three months I spent at the centre had a profound effect on me. At times I felt as if I was watching a documentary on TV, only this time was playing a leading role. There were patients who'd had severe head injuries, people recovering from stroke and brain tumours, in fact all manner of debilitating neurological problems. My eyes were opened to another world. I must briefly mention another significant development about this time. Whilst at Westminster Hospital I became very friendly with one of the nurses, so much so that when I'd finally left for the rehab. centre, this friendship had become a very unexpected romance. It's hard to measure the tremendous psychological lift this brought to bear in my continued recovery and optimistic, hopeful view of the world. By contrast the psychological and physical plight of many of my fellow patients who were coming to terms with their condition moved me more than anything I had ever experienced. The courage and determination shown by so many people, some very young and others around my own age, deeply affected me.

More than a few of these people at the same time as struggling to regain mobility were having to try to come to terms with lost marriages, loss of employment and loss of self-esteem. It angered me that there seemed to be no one in authority offering emotional support. I instinctively felt that just by listening in a positive way to their fears and hopes might offload some of the weight of these very real concerns. Not surprisingly many of my fellow patients were suffering from depression and melancholia; some, I'd discovered, had not been outside the centre for more than six or seven weeks mainly due to diminished confidence. Here was something I could take action on, so I organised a taxi one evening to take a few of us the mile or so to the local pub, so for a brief few moments changing our environment from clinical to social.

I believe that at this point, unknown to me at the time, seeds were being sown that would eventually lead me to where I am now, so maybe in retrospect I should give the Wolfson even more credit than I first realised, in not only getting me back literally on my feet again but playing a crucial role in starting me off on my vocational journey and leading me to enrol on a counselling course.

Early days in counselling training

I will summarise my personal development within the course learning community.

Throughout the course I found it helpful to try and simplify my learning – in other words to walk before I could run. An example of this was in my reading. Eager at first to read as much course-related literature as possible (mainly in the form of books) I slowly began to realise I was running ahead of myself. Without fully understanding or experiencing what I read I was leaving myself open to a sense of confusion and frustration. After deciding for a while to take a rest from looking at these books and to concentrate on looking at me and where I was I managed to see that I needed to relate to stimuli that were more at my level. This has been invaluable in understanding the course process more thoroughly and the need to trust and go through it even when disillusioned.

A back-to-basics approach in my learning appeared to be the best way forward and looking through my course journal I can pinpoint both moments of confusion and moments of clarity. Much of my confusion centred around the large group. I've struggled to look below what appeared to be going on at a surface level; perceived power struggles, as well as issues around gender, race and disability. All these were raised at some point in the course. This taught me that what I regarded as an issue hardly worth consideration was, for some, of major importance and showed me the importance of acquiring an empathetic understanding of my fellow students – not always easy – which I could then generalise to my work.

I often found that what happened in the group could be compared to what goes on in the wider world and that these processes can be viewed as taking place on political, social and personal levels. The key here is all about change, something I felt I was going through and would continue to go through if I were to realise my goal of becoming an effective counsellor. At times when the large group came together as a community there were periods of conflicting ideas and differing points of view, resulting in stalemate and silences, but through discussion and compromise we managed, sometimes painfully, to move forward as if the collective will of the community were at work. I confess to not always grasping fully how this came about. I could only perceive it, perhaps, as the total organism (which is the community) moving innately towards 'becoming', despite real or imagined hurdles. This was the toughest part of my development; smaller groups felt easier and more intimate.

Workshops gave me opportunities to look at counselling approaches I was unfamiliar with. Cognitive therapy, for instance, interested me at that time in that it appeared coherent and comprehensible and appealed to the practical side of my nature. Gestalt therapy is another approach I found exciting. Attending a day-long Gestalt workshop gave me an opportunity to experience the power of a particular technique familiar to many counsellors, the 'empty chair' technique. In this exercise I 'became' the assignment I had soon to write as part of my coursework. The experience of doing this was extremely helpful in allowing me to decide what shape the written assignment would take. Would I tape it or write it? I remember yelping in delight at the almost instantaneous result of the experiment, the clarifying effect was so simple, yet so effective. To become familiar with the many counselling models was necessary to shape my practice of counselling in general. It was important for me to explore these many approaches at my own pace however thirsty I was for more knowledge. It was vital that I didn't run ahead of myself and that I kept in mind the reassurance that everything I would need for my development would unfold in the due course of time.

My experience of being part of a self-directed course community was undoubtedly one of the most challenging endeavours I have ever undertaken. This way of learning (initially difficult even to get my head around) slowly and sometimes painfully showed me the many benefits attached to this model of learning. If I had to pick one of these many it would be that this way of learning – more precisely, this overall development on my part – is internalised in such a fashion as to become part of one's way of being, shaping, if you like, one's growing and changing attitude. To forget what one has learned in this way becomes almost as difficult as forgetting one's own name because it has become part of you and your interpersonal relationships with the course community. I feel a sense of truth in this knowledge, giving me the autonomy and self-confidence to succeed in this demanding line of work, also to become more self-directed in my life generally.

An example of my growing awareness can be found in that now I almost unconsciously find myself monitoring my feelings and behaviour. Ultimately this growing awareness has given me a greater insight and knowledge into where I am in relation to my work and my personal journey through life. I believe I am becoming a more perceptive and intuitive person, able to experience on a deeper level feelings that perhaps were once on the periphery of my awareness. The realisation that I have choice over my life's direction and am not merely a victim of circumstance is a tantalisingly liberating realisation. It is beginning to show me that the locus of evaluation or choice lies within me and that the only question that matters is 'Am I living in a way which is deeply satisfying to me, and which truly expresses me?' (Rogers 1961, p. 119). I may be some way from this state of being but simply to know that I am now on my way, brought about over two years on the course, leaves me with a greater sense of autonomy and self belief.

I would like to highlight some of the growth points that occurred for me during my formal training and how they relate to my working situation. The group process was the hardest part of the course for me. The dynamics at times surprised, distressed and amazed me. It felt at times as though we stagnated while at other times things appeared to move at an alarming pace. This showed me the need for flexibility and the need for a nurturing of mental energy. There were times when the large group moved from inactivity to what resembled a rollercoaster with the group becoming animated and vocal. There is no better example of this than during a plenary session at our second residential weekend. I remember the energy level soaring at one point when it appeared there were several things going on at the same time and as the level of energy climbed I felt it would never peak. I later noted that the atmosphere felt as if it was crackling with electricity. This group dynamic in effect acted as an energising factor in the group process and led us toward a more productive and flowing co-operation as we worked out and prioritised our learning for the forthcoming year. Indeed following the dynamics of this encounter it felt as if the group had entered a more harmonious relationship with itself and some of our best work was done in the second half of that particular weekend, culminating in an almost ritualistic bonding ceremony in the tranquil grounds of the All Saints Pastoral Centre where the weekend took place.

I learned the need to trust and nurture not only what is developing and growing within me but also within all the groups, both large and small, that I am part of. What I experience in such groups will help me in any future group work I become engaged in. There is a strong case for group therapy with people following stroke, especially persons with aphasia, who may have feelings of isolation. People can help each other to build confidence, which is so important in raising the spirit, thus speeding up the process of re-learning language again. The mere act of communicating, even non-verbally, has therapeutic benefits.

For me, working in the large group was at times a fearful experience, risky and oppressive. It was a case of feeling that fear and doing it anyway. I tried during the life of our group community to engage at some level with every course member. This I feel I achieved to a greater or lesser degree. There was a small handful of course members I never really got to know but, again, I am not sure it would have been possible to have worked at deeper levels with everyone over the two years anyway.

Was there anyone on the course I didn't like? This was a question I asked myself from time to time, especially during year one. The answer would come back as 'no' but certain members felt somewhat distanced from me maybe on a subconscious level. This was recognised at least by me and so in year two I made it a priority to try and work with these particular people in small groups, or one to one. During our second residential, I remarked that I would find it helpful to work with three course members I had had very little contact with in the previous year. When I did, in a learning group, any fear that we might not connect was quickly dispelled as we set about discussing the coming year's learning requirements for each of us and in an environment of mutual encouragement we gave each other that precious commodity: time. Time to explore and prioritise our needs for the coming year. We finished by commenting that we would find it useful to continue this group outside course time and although I later formed a stronger link with my old supervision group when the question of extra-curriculum groups was widened, I felt this encounter laid to rest any fantasies I may have had to do with future engagements on the course.

I feel my interpersonal skills have always been there and as my work pre-stroke was directly working with people and not machines, I have, over the years, developed these skills. The course helped focus and build on what was already in place. It is now easier for me to give and receive feedback in the knowledge that constructive criticism equals help that is helpful and gives me greater insight into how others view me. Feedback is invaluable in knowing more about oneself and letting more of yourself become known to others. Adopting a more open and non-defensive stance to others makes day-to-day exchanges a more pleasurable experience. I find this freer attitude encourages a similar response in others and invariably leads to more satisfying interpersonal relationships, also to franker, deeper, and more constructive communication with people in my counselling-related work and in every other area of my life. In short this approach helps make life just that little bit easier.

The two-year diploma course that I thought was pretty much all that was needed to gain an adequate understanding of what counselling is and what it means to give good, effective counselling has instead shown me that this was only the beginning of the process. Far from knowing what it's all about, I now see that this ongoing process will continue for the rest of my life; there will always be more to know and experience. Initially this realisation left me feeling somewhat deflated. Knowing that this area of work was an ongoing process of learning and change and I can never reach a stage where I can honestly say, 'I know it', led me to contemplate deeply on the implications and commitments of working in this field. My internal processes have begun to move me into viewing this prospect differently. I now see this as an exciting and challenging realisation, giving me infinite opportunities to change and grow on all levels. How wonderful to know there are continued and as yet unknown horizons for me to view in my journey of becoming.

There is a quiet pleasure in knowing that, by discovering more about me and my being, I create a reservoir of knowledge always available for use in my work. It stands to reason that the more I look inward, the more I discover and the more I discover, the more I know – and the more I can give of myself to my work and my clients.

A person-centred philosophy

There are many approaches to counselling that I find exciting and challenging but the one which I have explored deepest and most often, with which I was most familiar, and which felt most like me, was person-centred counselling. Carl R. Rogers (1902–87), the founder of person-centred counselling or psychotherapy, was influenced by many significant figures but always claimed above all, to be the student of his own experience and that of his clients and colleagues. In this simple acknowledgment lies an example of the refreshingly different approach to therapy that has made his work so innovative and demystifying. In the late 1920s he began to question the analytical approach to therapy in which he was schooled. Obviously this was risky. To go against the established ethos of diagnosis and interpretation exemplified by the likes of Freud risked being thought of as a heretic or, worse, a charlatan. None the less he remained true to his convictions. Here then is a perfect example of Rogers' 'organismic self' in action – that part of the self which houses the locus of evaluation, something Rogers places great emphasis on, so that doing what feels right proves to be 'a . . . trustworthy guide to behaviour' (Rogers 1961).

I like this attitude. My early impression of psychologists and others working in this field was that they were the experts, highly intelligent and powerful, and they had the answers. They appeared to cultivate this image, even to 'get off' on their feelings of superiority. Why one human being believes they know more about another's psychological make-up than the person themself and has the answers to their problems smacks to me of egotistic self-opinion and from the outset tips the scales of power away from the client and toward the therapist thereby confirming in the client a state of powerlessness. This is not conducive to growth and not likely to be either helpful or useful therapy. In contrast the person-centred approach is all about empowering the client. In the beginning this empowering can be frightening. Indeed, many clients would rather not have it, many are used to giving their power to parents, teachers, the state and so forth, falsely believing someone else knows what's best for them. They have in many cases completely lost touch with their organismic self and will not trust themselves to make valued judgments or decisions.

On the counselling course I experienced the fear and confusion of being handed my own power. I remember initially thinking: 'Great! Self-directed! Non-structured! That means no one tells you what to do – but if no one tells me what to do how will I learn?' This felt paradoxical, confusing. Soon I longed for direction, even just a little bit and so, slowly, my organismic self began to come into play. I began to listen, really listen, to myself, my needs and what I wanted to learn. Working with others developed my interpersonal skills, so that I gave and received what was necessary to achieve my aims. This was a hard discipline and remains so but the rewards have been boundless, ranging from increased self-confidence to a newly found humility, and it is from this humility that I say I haven't started to know what it truly entails to be an accomplished counsellor but I believe I have begun to.

I remember wondering when I decided to embark on training, whether I was academically capable of working in counselling. I'd left school with no real qualifications even though I'd enjoyed school immensely. It was reassuring to read on more than one occasion Rogers' statement that it is the counsellor's attitude to himself and his client, rather than his intellectual or theoretical ambitions, that are the most important factors in being an effective counsellor. It was his contention – and he held firm to it for over forty years – that if the counsellor is able to offer a facilitative climate where the core conditions for change and growth are present, this will almost certainly allow change to take place.

Three core conditions are fundamental to the person-centred counsellor. They are (1) congruence, realness or genuineness, (2) unconditional positive regard or total acceptance and (3) an empathetic understanding. It helps immensely to deliver these core conditions in a climate of warmth and kindness, as this gives the client a sense of being valued. As I become more confident in what I do and why I'm doing it I am finding a greater sense of self-love. This is essential: if you withhold such responses from yourself, warts and all, you can never genuinely offer that same acceptance, empathy and genuineness at the deepest level. You can be sure that clients will feel a falseness and will sense incongruity and deception. Plato said that there is nothing worse than self-deception, where the deceiver is always with you.

I have made it a goal in my work and my life to strive for the truth in every undertaking I pursue. This is not easily attained and needs constant monitoring and an ability to listen and know the self at a deep level. This works for me during spiritual healing, something I recommend as a facility in hearing the self. Reading Rogers, I have been struck by, amongst other things, a sense of kindness or tenderness and an openness that seems to come through in his writing. I can vouch for these qualities being therapeutic in their own right as very early on in my stay in hospital, when many health workers were busy attending to several patients at once and I felt vulnerable and confused and unable to speak, a simple smile or hand or even in a quieter moment, a few kind words, seemed to reach inside and touch me. Believe me when I say this free giving of kindness had the power to move me to the point of tears. Not of sorrow and certainly not of joy but I suppose of acknowledgment of my predicament. I remember such incidents almost nine years later, which is testament to their healing power. This experience was a lesson that has already been integrated in my own counselling. The unconditional kindness and respect shown to me helped me to see my own self-worth at a time when life and living had left me with a strong ambivalence regarding my future.

A story told by Rogers has become a favourite of mine and one I call on in moments of disillusionment. He tells of a boyhood memory of a potato bin that his parents kept in the basement of their house several feet below a small window. Despite the highly unfavourable conditions the potatoes would nevertheless begin to send out spindly pale white shoots groping towards the distant light of the window. Rogers compared these pathetic potatoes and their desperate struggle against all the odds with his many clients whose lives had been warped by circumstances and experiences, but who continued, nevertheless, with a directional or actualising tendency. Whether the environment is favourable or not, the behaviour of an organism, be it a plant or a human being, will tend toward a direction of maintaining, enhancing and reproducing itself. This potent constructive tendency is an underlying basis of the person-centred approach.

My own process of becoming has to continue if my work is to remain acceptable. This necessitates continually seeking to broaden my life experience, for without growth and development of my self I am unlikely to be able to facilitate the same in my clients. My task must always be to create new conditions for the client. The analogy of the potato lends itself nicely here in that the task is to provide a rich and nutritious soil and a different climate in which the client can recover from trauma or distress and begin to flourish and grow as the unique individual he or she actually is. I am struck by what an impact Rogers' writings, thought and indeed his whole philosophy have had on me. Here is someone who has taught me so much and helped shape my thinking through his clarity of thought and expression. I admire greatly his ability to communicate on all levels and his overriding belief in the innate goodness of the human organism. All this from someone I haven't as yet even seen a picture of! It may sound somewhat pretentious (I hope it doesn't come across like that) but I count him as a true friend, for when I read his works I get a real sense that he is talking exclusively to me.

Reliving the stroke: a Gestalt exercise

In the course of learning about Gestalt therapy, members of my group were invited to write an account of the most significant episode in our lives, as if it was happening to us in the here and now and using the first person. I chose to write an account of my stroke:

> This feels wrong, scary, why can I not feel my right side, my right arm get up move around it's my circulation shit I can't stand up must get to the phone Oh God I can't speak these are not words I must keep trying don't hang up it's me Harry for fuck's sake help yes yes an ambulance get to the front door what on earth is happening the cat is real this must be real what's happening to me? Ambulance men I can't speak how do I know where the fucking key is? Who's going to feed the cat? Oh fuck what's happened to me?

> You're the doctor, you tell me I can't speak this is weird shit Toots she'll starve.

> Alan, where did he come from? I don't know what happened I can't speak you have to feed Toots I know I must gesture my arm's dead I'll point to my mouth act like a cat come on Al cat cat cat yes feed the fucking cat. Who did what to me? Must sleep must hide too many questions what on earth is happening?

> Stroke. Me. How why when walk talk, arm hand oh shit wheelchair. Useless fucking doctor I'll show you I'll be out of here in two weeks. Speaking must learn speaking therapy speech therapy first then walk then arm.

> Shit I've been here almost a month I'm not getting better my best friend's a wheelchair something's missing another therapy? I'm scared will I get better? Lots of visitors no one to talk to can't talk properly speech therapist must make her listen shit I'm in deep trouble can't hide look at me for fuck's sake hear me can't you understand. Push everything off her desk yes phone books pads paper the lot. Now look at me yes I'm frightened what will happen to me it's hurting inside listen to me please help me God help me!

> Can't even read properly that word says stroke urgh that word can't read the rest my turn for physio can't fucking walk beautiful nurses lovely physiotherapists uniforms sex can I? Information please no one to speak to I mean really speak to.

> Hey I can sort of read the stroke poster can you visit someone who's had a stroke call Stroke Association. God! If you give me back my voice let me walk I'll visit people is it a deal? I don't think God works

like that or does he God if you can't help me then piss off and leave me alone. One step, I walked one step, did you see that one step. I can walk, must work harder, I can fucking walk!

The Wolfson Rehabilitation Centre, this is the place, this is where I'll make my big recovery. I'll miss Westminster, shit, three months, I'm getting better slowly I am getting better my speech is pretty good no more no's when I mean yes still slow but no more speech therapy must get rid of this fucking wheelchair, I'm getting better must work harder must walk again. Pippa the nurse says she'll visit me hope so she's been a great help things are looking up.

Oh! God it feels like I'm watching a documentary on television, only I'm in this one, shit what happened to him, brain tumour, car crash, this is another world, where's the help this guy's a mess, scars, stitches, medication, why's his head so big? Wife's left, no home, no job, I'll bring him down the pub, six weeks in this place give him a break Don't worry about your head wear a hat we'll get a cab.

This place is unbelievable so much sadness so much courage so much spirit so much humour thank God for humour I'll never forget this place or the people here I feel like one of the lucky ones 'cos I'm still getting better still working hard must keep working hard.

Time to close for Christmas I won't be coming back here Jesus my stroke was in June and now it's almost Christmas I've still a long way to go. Must go back to Westminster become an outpatient still need more physio still making progress slowly so slow I'm told recovery can go on for two years or more must keep working pushing.

Spiritual healing is helping more than I realise glad I listened it's been good advice lifting me powerful stuff.

Where to now why was there no one to talk to why is there still no one to talk to about feelings emotions the future the past. The physiotherapists agree suggesting maybe I could do it instead of moaning where's that poster what about my deal with God – spiritual healing. Yes of course I can do that I can talk almost as well as I used to I can walk and I'm still improving I'd be good at it I could be a counsellor. Hillsborough. *The Marchioness* and King's Cross all these disasters had counsellors stroke is a disaster as well it should have counselling too that's what I'll do a two-week counselling course that should do the trick now where do they hold counselling courses?

As I write this I smile at my naïvety back then, in thinking I could crack counselling in two weeks! Writing this account in the first person, of the most significant episode in my life so far, a typical Gestalt exercise, was a powerful experience. I found myself entering into the feelings, thoughts, emotions. I felt again, albeit it in a rather diluted manner, the fear, confusion and hopelessness and this reliving of the experience was at times alarming. Also during the exercise I recalled that while in hospital I tried to explain to a friend that it felt as if my left leg was mocking my right leg's early attempts to gain some mobility. Eventually this mockery was replaced by a softening, almost supportive stance, as if showing the other how it's done. I now recognise this as an early example of a Gestalt perspective in which different parts of the body engage in a dialogue with each other and it's funny to think I was using Gestalt before I even knew it.

Starting work at City Dysphasic Group (CDG)

In January 1995 I began working as a part-time counsellor at CDG which is a therapy centre and support group for people with long term aphasia. It goes without saying how significant this was for me as the original aim of my training was to eventually become a full-time paid counsellor allowing me to come off state benefits. This was to be the final act in my long journey of recovery and developing a new self-identity. I had many thoughts and feelings as the time grew nearer for me to take up my position at the Department of Clinical Communication Studies, City University. I was excited at the prospect of 'going to work' although this excitement was tinged with more than a little apprehension, but I knew that in the right supportive environment I would continue to grow as a counsellor. I had met with staff and colleagues and was made to feel welcome. I had discussed my role with the Clinic Director and had been shown my counselling room where I would be offering my service to dysphasic clients attending the Department as well as to partners and relatives who were indirectly affected by dysphasia. There was also the potential for extending this service to staff and speech and language therapy students. Two-and-a-half years on I am pleased to report my ongoing development has continued along the path towards becoming an effective stroke and dysphasia counsellor. On both my working days I have a full caseload of four clients on each day, roughly divided between clients who attend CDG and outside referrals mostly coming from speech and language therapists from health authorities in or around London. I am also seeing more partners of dysphasic clients often together with their dysphasic partners and there has been a steady increase in student therapists. This last client group is, I believe, a result of the culture of the Department, where recognising a need for personal counselling is seen as more of a strength than as a weakness.

Disability

I would like to discuss the wider social context in which my counselling takes place. As a person with a disability, the question of equal opportunities is something that directly affects me. I have always addressed this issue in an open and honest manner and while it's OK to be as aware of the possible disadvantages some people may have as a result of disability, race, gender etc., I have found that ultimately it is the job of the individual concerned to raise any issues or concerns he/she may have around this sometimes emotive issue if they feel their needs are not being met. As I become clearer about why I do what I do, I try to keep at the centre of my being my original reasons for embarking on this path. I believe I have turned around something that I initially perceived as a disadvantage and now use it to my advantage. I believe the person who is perceived as socially disadvantaged needs to be encouraged to adopt a positive self-image, something I'm becoming more skilled at facilitating, despite the varying complexities of each new client I come in contact with. So much depends on the client's social perceptions before the disability was acquired and the amount of self-motivation, which can be greatly enhanced by the client's immediate family and friends acting in as supportive a way as possible. I feel I should mention at this point the trauma many partners and family are faced with at the sudden adjustment of family roles. Speaking as a man this forced role change can be one of the most distressing aspects of a newly acquired disability as unfortunately many men are not socialised to ask for help and are generally expected to be in control of themselves and their situation. It's no wonder that the social fabric of the whole family can be put under sudden and tremendous stress.

This is where I try to use my whole self or my 'unique' self if you like, in the counselling process. As someone who has personally experienced a sudden catastrophic situation in the form of a stroke and recovered sufficiently, I have at my disposal visible evidence to support my message of hope, valuable as often hopelessness is among the first feelings to set in for the person who has newly acquired a disability.

Many individuals are viewed by others as disabled but do not consider themselves to be disabled. How one views oneself is the all-important factor. For instance, I do not consider myself as disabled most of the time. It's when I need to, say, run for a bus and find I can no longer do this that my personal disability is brought home to me. Acceptance is the key word here. If I fully accept that I'll have to wait for the next bus, I have in that instance overcome my disability at least on a cognitive level. Thus, a person with a disability may not be handicapped in certain roles or environments. Another key word is 'limitation'. The famous violinist Itzhak Perlman, who is mobility impaired, is not handicapped in his role as a violinist, although he would be handicapped as, say, a soccer player. In my counselling work I try to focus on what the person can, rather than cannot, do to build on the existing personality and so I encourage the individual not to dwell on limbs that may not function, but rather to look at the self as a whole person. Of course to ignore the impairment would be dangerously inappropriate as this could help the person to deny the problem, often a consequence of a sudden disability. Until denial is overcome, the patient can never move towards an acceptance of what has occurred.

I would like at this point to say a little about a subject that for many people can be a little embarrassing, but none the less is a crucial issue – sex. That most basic of instincts and the concerns around it, are often not given the very necessary attention they deserve. Again I draw on personal experience to verify this. After struggling to come to terms with the medical consultant's totally insensitive explanation of what had happened to me and his non-committal response to questions, more and more concerns surfaced. I was left feeling that life had all but ceased for me. Among these many concerns was one in particular, one I really didn't want to confront for fear of the answer being negative and as I looked around for somewhere or someone to bring these fears to, I realised my options were few. I like to think I have no great problem in discussing male sexuality or sex in general in a mature manner, with members of the opposite sex, but at a time of crisis, with very poor speech and low self-esteem, it was a different matter. All the nurses, physiothera-pists and occupational therapists were female, as was my speech therapist. Whether they too were embarrassed to broach the subject or whether they didn't see it as an issue I don't know, but for me it was of paramount importance and the longer it remained unad-dressed the more anxious I became. During this time the very word 'paralysis' took on even more sinister connotations than it ought and my imagination, left unchecked, was free to indulge in spurious thoughts and feelings.

After roughly two weeks, my body's own post-shock healing process was beginning to get under way and the gradual return of normal basic bodily functions was heralded with the most welcome reintroduction of my libido. This allowed me to dispel at least one fear for the future but it left me thinking 'Why didn't anyone tell me?'

Here was a real concern that need not have even been an issue. Had I been a woman, there would have been a wealth of opportunity to address any worries I had about sexual function, as the health workers surrounding me were almost exclusively female.

This leads me to the male gender role, which appears to play a significant part in a man's adjustment to a disability. Our society's expectations for men make it more difficult for them to be disabled (Skord and Schumacher 1982). Liss-Levinson (1982) states that 'the traditional male sex role dictates that men are rational, independent, and capable of handling any and all crises. Men are . . . expected to be healthy, vigorous, strong and sexually rapacious.' After sudden disability, many of the roles a man is accustomed to playing become challenged or compromised, leaving him feeling he has lost control of his life. This loss of control is made worse by the disabled man's sudden dependency, this dependency being in contrast with society's image of the self-sufficient male.

For four years I attended a support group at Westminster Social Services once a week, specifically for men with disabilities. I had ample opportunity to explore with others many of these issues and learned much from my encounters in the group which gave me a greater understanding of the wider social context in which my counselling takes place. Much of what I have written on this particular point has related to men. In the past I have had many female clients and although I feel I would be able talk about sexual matters with women, so far this has not been necessary to any great degree. As the majority of counsellors are women I feel I have a real contribution to make around this area of counselling, in balancing the ratio, thus offering a wider choice overall.

Part of my counselling is, in some cases, to offer hope of a return to work. This entails use of myself, not so much as a role model, but to show that despite the onset of a disability, it is still possible to make a worthwhile contribution to society. Of course this is not always as simple as it sounds and depends on the severity of the disability, but here again the main thrust of my counselling is to facilitate a climate of hope by concentrating in a positive way on the new choice of options that may be available – in short to endeavour to bring to bear for the client a climate of self-worth. Ultimately, the disabled person (man or woman) does not want to be treated like a disabled person. They want to be treated as an individual. I have not yet focused on class, race and religion, indeed I may be politically naïve in some of these matters. That is for me to rectify through a continued awareness of these issues and an appreciation of their significance, not only for me but for my future clients in this ever-changing society.

The emotional sequelae of stroke range from fear, anxiety and irritability to emotional lability, anger, frustration and depression. These emotional changes may be compared to those after bereavement. As one who has been through this process, I can testify to this as true; some of these emotional changes were. for me, anyway, fairly fleeting whilst others were more deep-seated and therefore harder to overcome. Because everyone who has an acquired disability is a unique individual, the process is never exactly the same but can be viewed as a four-stage adaptation process: anxiety is the first stage and during this time the person requires reassurance and help in focusing in the present. He/she needs to be encouraged to keep up with speech if necessary, physio and occupational therapy. This is important as most physical recovery in stroke is made within the first and second year, so the need to start early with all therapies cannot be stressed enough. The second stage is accommodation, a time for reconciliation to differences and realisation of a changing lifestyle. The third stage (which for me occurred around 18 months post stroke) is assimilation. This stage centres on growth, challenge and change. It is true to say assimilation continues throughout life. The fourth and final stage – reflux, may not occur at all. I personally haven't experienced this. It can happen at any time and is a regression to an earlier stage due to a serious physical, emotional or financial difficulty. Successful adaptation requires a reworking of all subsequent stages. It is necessary to have a clear understanding of these stages of adaptation as this helps to facilitate more effective counselling. In my case, unfortunately my understanding of these stages comes from my own experience and most of us learn best, really learn, from our own experience. Confucius puts it well: 'I hear and I forget, I see and I remember, I do and I understand'. Knowledge of the aforementioned stages helps any therapist to focus on the client's needs more specifically and to know where they are emotionally. Another element that plays a major role in the healing process is that of spiritual healing. This powerful form of healing has put me more in touch with my spiritual self and given me a deeper understanding of this part of the human organism. I believe this is where the central truth, the core of a person is housed. This has been a gradual and exciting realisation on my part and I aim to continue developing the spiritual element of my counselling work. To give a clearer picture of what I mean here, if we view the human spirit as a flame, it is as if this flame were almost extinguished following a serious accident or illness. In my counselling, I aim to rekindle and nurture this flame. This is essential as it is widely believed amongst professional health care workers that there is a strong relationship between emotional wellbeing and physical recovery.

Plato said 'Never attempt to heal the body, until you first heal the mind'. With due deference I would add 'and spirit'. This holistic approach serves to offer the client/ patient the maximum opportunity of a fuller recovery. To summarise then, the four-stage adaptation process requires the use of various counselling skills. If these skills are used accurately and effectively the overall outcome will be that the client will accept themselves and make the necessary adjustments needed to carry on their life. They will re-establish roles in their personal, social and family life and, if the client and family are flexible, the future for the client as a contributor to the family will be assured. In my work many clients have been left with varying degrees of speech problems following a stroke. Experiencing dysphasia personally has given me an insight into this distressing condition and my aim is to use this insight to its maximum positive effect in my work.

Difficulties

Now that the structure of the counselling service is in place, I would like to describe some of the aspects of my work that I have found difficult from a practical viewpoint. I had, in my counselling training, worked hard on my personal growth through careful exploration of my own attitudes, beliefs and values as well as my prejudices. Together with a gradual understanding of the counselling process and acquisition of practical counselling skills, I felt I had adopted a professional attitude to my counselling work with clients. However the side of my work I had not given the same consideration to was the organisational and administrative aspect of running a counselling service. In many ways my work prior to my stroke had not called for these skills and very soon I discovered that organising myself efficiently regarding referrals, returning phone enquiries, waiting lists etc. was a discipline that did not come easily. I know the importance of keeping notes after every counselling session and see that as an extension of my work that helps to clarify and detail the actual counselling process.

Changing from counsellor role into a secretarial/administrator role challenged my flexibility. I have become more skilled at this important aspect of my work through careful and ongoing monitoring and together with practical support from colleagues, and I now find I am more comfortable with this role. These administration skills are necessary in the implementation of referrals. This usually begins with a phone call from a speech therapist enquiring about the service, who it is available to and what the procedure is. In general, I will see anyone who has been affected by stroke and/or dysphasia, the only stipulations are that the proposed client has personally asked for counselling, is medically stable (as we have no nursing facilities) and can get to CDG under their own steam. I will ask for a referral letter detailing relevant information. When the referrer offers their own opinions on the client's issues or needs, I strive to prevent any prior assumptions from allowing me to receive a new client with anything other than an open mind. Another's opinion, however well intended, is exactly that – another opinion.

The counselling process

The importance of creating the three core conditions of congruence, empathy and unconditional positive regard is a fundamental part of my work; indeed my overall aim is to continue to develop and maintain such attitudes not only in my work, but in my life as a whole. Perhaps this will necessitate me not only adopting these qualities, but instead striving to become them. It has been said 'The counsellor can only go as far with the client as the counsellor can go with him/her self. What therapists find in themselves, they can recognise in others.' In other words my ongoing personal development underpins the development of my ethical and conceptual framework of counselling. An ongoing commitment to the client can be made through understanding myself and my counselling role. As this commitment implies, the client's welfare is of paramount importance. That said, the importance of professional boundaries and their implementation have always to be to the fore. Although each of these boundaries matters in its own right, confidentiality ranks high in my estimation, as this, and punctuality (starting and ending on time), will enable trust and continuity to develop in the counselling relationship. Being consistently aware of these boundaries contributes to maintaining a healthy therapeutic relationship and helps to avoid giving the client my own issues, if and when they occur. Continually monitoring this awareness helps also in recognising what the client's issues may throw up for me during the counselling process, as many of my past and future clients will have suffered strokes. This awareness is essential if I'm to avoid becoming lost in the process and to recognise incidents of transference and counter-transference when they occur. In ensuring these distorting reactions are given full attention, supervision will and does play an important role in my ethical framework of counselling.

Broadly speaking, my aims of therapy are to identify areas of difficulty with the client – these may be varied for some clients and for others they may be unclear. It will often take several sessions before clear aims become apparent. Where these are established and realised as attainable we have a framework within which the client can then work towards these aims or goals. In many respects, the initial session is the most important as trust needs to be established in the relationship as early as possible; many clients will feel anxious and, for many, seeing a 'counsellor' is yet another unfamiliar experience following their illness. My first priority therefore is to convey a sense of calm in the counselling room, my pacing will be unhurried, hopefully indicating a certain freedom and space to breathe. This can help me as much as the client and I may even comment on the fact that counsellors can get anxious too. I may suggest some simple controlled breathing exercises if that feels appropriate. My overall aim in these early moments in the relationship is for the client to feel as safe and as comfortable as possible in order that they are best able to begin to say, or communicate, what has brought them to see me. This is also a time for discussing the preferred means of communication, which can be verbal or non-verbal depending on the degree of difficulty or a mixture using writing, drawing, painting or gesture. In my experience, it is not the client's lack of speech that tends to create any lasting difficulties in our developing relationship, but the client's ability to fully understand what is being said to them. It is this that will challenge the effectiveness of counselling.

By the end of the initial session, it is my hope that the client will leave feeling that someone has listened and really heard them. Carl Rogers wrote in his book *A Way of Being* (1980) that during counselling sessions when clients know that they have really been heard at a deep and empathetic level, they will often be moved to tears. This is my experience, in some sense these may be tears of joy and relief as though the client were saying 'Thank God somebody heard me. Somebody knows what it is like to be me.' It is by periodically checking that I am fully understanding what the client is communicating, maintaining the unhurried air in the dialogue, hearing the meanings as well as the words and sharing, if it feels helpful, my own feelings, that the client will feel able to use further sessions to explore issues and feelings that maybe painful or frightening.

At some point in the developing relationship, a client often asks about my own personal experience of stroke and dysphasia. This can be an important moment. I am always aware that the client's needs are paramount and that any disclosure on my part must be given with this in mind. However, my disclosure can be an opportunity to develop a level of intimacy and openness that will, I hope, enable the client to move forward in their exploration of their own issues. It is also my hope that by sharing my own experience of the fear, confusion and anger I experienced following my stroke, my client will feel it permissible and safe to do likewise. Because of this my personal experience of stroke is a unique strength that can be invested in my work with clients.

Loss is a recurring theme for almost all clients. Careful explanation of the grieving process to the client, who may be unfamiliar with the term, can be helpful in allowing exploration of the stages of grief and often leads to the client recognising where they are in this process.

I find it useful near the end of a session to briefly summarise what has been discussed in the session and whenever possible I will offer some positive feedback. Generally the duration of counselling will be determined by periodically reviewing our work together. At all times I ensure that the client does not feel pressurised – many people recovering after stroke report feeling rushed from one therapy to another by busy therapists. My overall aim will be to assist the client with the identification and clarification of their issues through exploration of feelings and emotions in the hope that this will lead to a greater awareness of choices or options for the future. It is my hope that by the end of counselling there will be a change in the client's attitude towards their enforced change of circumstance. This will be assisted by the quality of the relationship that has grown between us over a series of sessions. This relationship will have trust and a sense of safety for the client and therefore allow for a degree of confrontation. Confrontation in a counselling sense will often allow the client to view his or her situation from a different perspective and can encourage or motivate the client to move nearer to some level of acceptance or resolution. Without confrontation the client may stick at some stage in the grieving process or may recognise and identify which stage they are at, yet not be able to find solutions to these.

Ending therapy

The decision to end therapy will largely be made by spending time reviewing the progress that has been or is being made in our sessions. The aims that were discussed earlier to some extent will have guided our work together and through resolution and raised awareness the client may feel ready to explore the options and choices that are open to them. The focus may be on viewing achievable goals in the client's personal and social life and what resources are available to him or her that may assist in implementing them. In some sense the effectiveness of a series of counselling sessions cannot be truly known until a client has spent a period or time assimilating the process they have undergone. I will always leave an option for the client to return at any time if they feel it would be helpful to review their progress.

Supervision

I have known my supervisor for as long as I first began thinking about enrolling on an introductory counselling course. The quality of our relationship and its continued growth has been invaluable to me over the years – in particular it helps in allowing me to monitor my own process with clients. My supervisor's background as a psychodynamic counsellor is useful in giving me a different view as to what may be taking place in me on an unconscious level when I work with clients. It has helped me to recognise and separate my own needs from those of the client, an especially valuable insight that still requires continual monitoring. Supervision is an ongoing opportunity for growth and self-awareness. In my early work with clients it seemed that I was often guided by the need to appear 'professional' coupled with a need to feel I was 'doing it right'. This could be put down to inexperience or self-doubt, but acknowledging it and bringing it to my awareness led to further insights such as a need in me for my clients to 'feel better', a need to get results. These were my needs and certainly had no place in the counselling room. Supervision allowed for the exploration of the significance and validity of these needs and continues to be an insightful and clarifying experience. Indeed, supervision and experience have been instrumental in changing my need to 'do it right' into allowing myself more and more just to be.

Spirituality

Since my stroke I have become aware of a spiritual dimension within me. This realisation was brought about, I believe, as a reaction to my stroke and has been enhanced and maintained by self-development work on counselling courses and by continued encounters in my current work. Close friends are witness to this phenomenon as greater spiritual awareness led me to seek spiritual healing some 18 months after my illness. I'm pretty quiet these days about the effect that these powerful and therapeutic encounters engendered in me. I would go so far as to say the path I am now on was revealed to me during a series of healing sessions in which answers to barely formed questions seemed to become clear and obvious. This clarity of thought contrasts greatly with my then confused state of mind and growing feelings of despair about my place and purpose in this world. At the heart of my distress lay questions that struck at the very core of my existence – Who am I? What am I? Why am I? I suppose that in many ways I had lost who I was and was struggling to find or regain a sense of self. Was it then coincidence that within days of receiving spiritual healing which I had been extremely sceptical about to begin with, I began to feel such a strong and real sense of purpose, so strong that for a while it scared me? It was impossible though to be scared of a feeling that was so overwhelmingly positive and energising. These very real and uplifting feelings left me feeling quite literally amazed. It is difficult to articulate these experiences, some may feel it too esoteric to have any substance. I believe internal and external experiences during my rehabilitation were leading me toward what I now do, only this was obscured by a fear of the future and confusion which weighed me down. Spiritual healing was the powerful catalyst that lifted me above the negativity which had grown within me and began to show me what I had to do to fulfil my potential and thereby my destiny. I have been told, and believe, that everyone has an ability to heal in some form or another. By acknowledging this universal ability and allowing a healing presence to emerge within the counselling relationship through genuine and unreserved communication, another dimension can be brought to bear in the therapeutic relationship. Healing is a reality and through embracing and accepting this reality, I have found that at certain times and with certain clients with whom a deep connection has developed, healing energy has been released. I experience this release as a flow of warmth, closeness and love which by the end of the session leaves me energised and uplifted, together with a sense of humility and privilege at having been allowed to share in a client's often painful and vulnerable view of their world. This section of the chapter has, in many respects, been the most difficult for me to express as the subject is an abstract one, but I do hope it gives a feel for the existential quality of dialogue that can be present when real contact between two people has been established, the outcome of which can be a gradual releasing of the client's innate ability to self-heal.

Today and tomorrow

An exciting aspect of my work that has developed over the last year
and a half is facilitating discussions with speech and language therapy students on such topics as loss, anger and depression. Two
colleagues, Chris Ireland and Sue Boazman, and myself, all counsellors with personal experience of dysphasia, have put together basic
counselling skills workshops which have been extremely well
received. It is through these workshops and discussions and the offer
of a counselling supervision and advice service to students, that the
culture of the Department as a whole is aiming to promote a good
model of practice, challenging traditional attitudes to disability that
often see the person with a disability as a helpless victim. The philosophy and practice of the Department is to enable and support clients
through a social model of disability that focuses on clients living with
their disability.

In concluding this chapter my plans for future work and personal
development continue to excite and challenge me. Having
completed a part-time Gestalt counselling skills course at the Gestalt
Centre in London last year, I have gained a basic understanding of
this more dynamic approach to counselling with its emphasis on
awareness and working in the here and now, complementing my
Rogerian grounding. Recently, I have become interested in personal
construct therapy and am hoping to take an extensive course in the
not-too-distant future.

As I stated earlier, although when I began my training my overall
objective was to get back into full-time employment, I have slowly
begun to change my views on this. For the most part I find being a
stroke counsellor stimulating and rewarding, however, occasionally I
have been aware of feeling emotionally drained and under strain. I
now recognise that to be satisfied with the quality of work I offer is
more important than the quantity. Indeed one of the most important
things I have learnt since I began my counselling work was my own
limitations regarding a 'comfortable workload' and to work within
this comfort zone. The evolving variety of other aspects of my work
have helped immensely here – giving talks, running discussions, even
writing this chapter have all contributed to create an overall balance
in my work. This variety in turn sustains my excitement and enthusiasm by stretching and stimulating me and thereby attending to my
own need for personal satisfaction and self-esteem.

I sometimes amaze myself when I contemplate the path life has
taken me down since that fateful June day. It feels almost as if some

celestial force, something bigger, more powerful, had preordained that this be so and the first part of me to get this message or instruction was my organismic self which innately knew what was needed to enhance my potential and growth with its positive and trustworthy messages. As a result, instead of losing trust in the process of life I have turned this real-life nightmare around into an embracing of life and what it still has to offer. I could not have foreseen my life's direction from my hospital bed in the early days of my recovery and on reflection I do not think I could have dared hope for an outcome so positive and rewarding. I have mentioned the role that loss often plays in the process of recovery and resolution and feel able to report that I have gained far more in my life from my stroke than I feel I have physically lost. While I very much wish I had never personally experienced stroke and its residual problems, the stark reality is I did, but through a process of listening to and trusting my organismic self, I have been able to enrich my life through a choice of work that affords me opportunities for continued growth and self-actualisation. My earnest hope for the future is to help facilitate clients in this very same process.

Chapter 6
Lost child: therapeutic work with a mother of an infant with severe learning disabilities

KATHRYN S LEWIS

Introduction – the referral – measurement issues – observations of mother and child – emerging themes during counselling – progress in the mother–infant relationship – a new daughter – ethical issues – summary – conclusions.

The clinical case study presented here was begun at the time when I was attending a one-year course at the Tavistock Clinic in London entitled 'psychodynamic work in learning disability'. The course attracts people from numerous professions who have contact with learning-disabled children and adults, and aims to facilitate a wider understanding of these clients and their families from a psychodynamic perspective. The intention is not to train people to become psychoanalytical psychotherapists but to enhance and extend the considerable skills and training that each individual brings with him or her. As such, clinical psychologists, psychiatrists, nursing staff, social workers, art therapists, dance therapists, residential care managers, and other professionals come together to share the nature of their work and enrich one another's understanding of the dilemmas and difficulties faced from a developing psychodynamic perspective. The clinical work carried out in the case presented below has been influenced greatly, therefore, by the knowledge and understanding taken away from this training.

Introduction

People with severe physical and cognitive disabilities discern at a very early stage that they can provoke many uncomfortable, negative emotions in others. The dawning of this realisation often begins with what Donald Winnicott described as the first mirror of a mother's eyes. Sinason (1992, p. 276) commented:

> As babies we look up into the eyes of our primary carer and in that shiny mirror we see how loved we are. We do not ask 'Mirror mirror on the wall, who is the fairest of them all?' That is when rivalry begins or when the mirror tells the tale of those not loved for what is inside them. No, the first mirror tells us whether we were wanted, whether there is a real space for us; whether we are thought to be the most wonderful new thing in the world.

It is from this mirror that we gain a sense of self; an internal image of who we are and how others perceive us. If a child is not wanted then the image reflected back is painfully negative. Sinason (1992, p. 277) commented further that the mirror does not have to be a visual one:

> Blind children who cannot see the look in their parents' eyes can hear the tone of voices, feel the response of bodies and receive back an image of worth or worthlessness.

As such, infants with disabilities may have coldness, shame, fear, guilt or anger mirrored back to them in their early interactions with a mother grieving the loss of her perfectly formed fantasy child (Raphael-Leff 1993). For some children, the effort to survive is too great in the face of rejection and they may die an emotional death or succumb to an illness resulting in physical death. The bond between mother and child when seen in this light is, therefore, potentially life-saving as well as life-giving. Sinason (1992) has pointed out, however, that parents are frequently not given adequate emotional support in the early period so that the bonding process is at best delayed for some time and at worst fails completely.

When the degree of disability in the child is severe, perhaps because of multiple disabilities, the relationship is frustrated further by the child's struggle to maintain a physiological and psychological equilibrium resulting in protracted development of sucking, reciprocal smiling, play, and other attachment-enhancing behaviours (Als 1982). Moreover, if depression is present in the mother, she has fewer resources for encouraging the relationship with her compromised infant and a vicious downward spiral of negative responsiveness on both sides may result. Indeed, depressed mothers tend to be unresponsive to infant behaviour, tending to be either withdrawn, or intrusive and hostile (Cohn et al. 1986). It is understandable, therefore, that many mothers find it enormously difficult to bond with a child under such circumstances.

In addition to the difficulties just described, there may be what Selma Fraiberg described as 'ghosts in the nursery', the 'visitors from the unremembered past of parents, the uninvited guests at the christening' (Fraiberg 1980). Brazelton and Cramer (1991, p. 139) commented:

> The parents are unable to react to the infant's signals, because they are busy communicating with a ghost. This ghost may occupy the whole space, leaving no chance for the parents to see their child, or it may interfere with specific issues: eating, sleeping, discipline. The ghost's intrusion thus reveals a corresponding vulnerability in the parent's past.

During my own work with parents of children with disabilities, there have been numerous examples of such 'ghosts' from the past. One case involved a mother of a young child with epilepsy and learning difficulties. When Peter had a seizure, Barbara would become extremely anxious and would run away into another room. During the night, if she heard his body banging against the gate on his bed, she would put the bedclothes over her head so that she could not hear him. Although she had an ambivalent relationship with her son, Barbara's ultimate fear was that Peter would die. When encouraged to reflect further on her anxieties about the seizures, Barbara gave a vivid account of Peter sitting up in his bed swaying around seeming unable to recognise anyone. During the same session, Barbara reported that her father had died because of a brain tumour when she was 14 years old so she was encouraged to talk about the memories of him during the later stages of his illness. Barbara became tearful and said that she loved her father but they had a difficult relationship. When she visited him in hospital, he did not seem to recognise her at all and had a glazed, distant look. In retrospect, she felt angry and sad that they were not able to say goodbye. The family had encouraged Barbara not to attend the funeral and afterwards she felt unable to talk about him because her mother would become extremely upset. Over the years, she learned to put him to the back of her mind because of the painful feelings evoked and the process of mourning (see Worden 1991) was therefore never completed. Barbara was enabled to make the link between her experiences of Peter's seizures and the impression of her father just before he died. She began to realise that she had projected some of the powerful feelings about the relationship with her father onto her son and that the 'ghost' of her father, who was apparent whenever Peter had a seizure, revived the agony of the loss. Barbara was able to begin the process of mourning the loss of her father, and was able to acknowledge and understand some of the mixed feelings about her son and his disabilities. Her anxieties reduced to the point where she could tolerate Peter's seizures without flying into a desperate avoidance strategy.

In a similar vein, Sinason (1992, p. 325) gave another example of this dynamic known as projective identification:

> . . . one deprived woman battered her baby when it cried. She could not bear the cry because she felt it was her own. Everything dependent and fragile in her that she could not bear had been projected into the baby. The baby's cries were then intolerable.

A further example from my own clinical work is of a mother with a child who sustained a head injury in a road traffic accident as an infant. George was a challenging boy because he had severe learning disabilities, hearing impairment, and associated difficulties in receptive and expressive communication. As such, he needed a fair amount of one-to-one support in order to remain occupied and content. He would seek attention from his exhausted parents constantly and sometimes would do things repeatedly that he knew were unacceptable even though this would make his parents angry. His mother, Vicky, reported that at times she would shout and scream at George when she was at 'the end of her tether'. However, if her partner, Dean, shouted at him, she would jump to his defence immediately and sometimes this would undermine Dean's attempts to set limits on George's behaviour. When encouraged to reflect on the underlying anxieties about her behaviour in this respect, Vicky began to talk about the relationship with her own father. Vicky's father was a man who tended to fly into rages and on a number of occasions, physically assaulted her mother. She lived in constant fear of his anger and felt helpless and lonely. Vicky was able to learn that she had identified with her disabled son through the helpless, frightened, child part of herself whenever her partner became angry. When she defended her son, she was defending herself as a little girl who had no one to make her feel safe.

During a later session, Vicky reported that she had stopped undermining her partner's attempts to set limits with George and they had started to use some behaviour management advice that had reduced the number of occasions when either parent would blow up. Brazelton and Cramer (1991, p. 158) point out that such projective processes are part of normal functioning:

> For a mother to become attuned to her infant's needs, she must rely on an identification with parts of her own infantile experience, now projected onto the baby. At the same time, if she is to learn about her baby (experiencing true mutuality), the mother needs also to 'pull back' from this identification and respect the infant's objective, individual signals.

Stokes (1987) described another kind of projection which is apparent in the general population but is often found in families where there is an individual with a disability. In such cases, individuals can split off and disown unacceptable parts of themselves and project them into the child so that 'the handicapped child can become the receptacle for all the handicapped and stupid parts of every member of the family'. Brazelton and Cramer (1991, p. 213) expanded on this point:

> The child is cast in the role of scapegoat of the family; he or she is used to focus and represent the 'bad' characteristics of other family members. Each person projects inner feelings of inadequacy onto him; the visible defect serves to materialise the evidence of badness, yet protects the self-esteem of the other family members. Self-fulfilling prophecies then accentuate the child's potential for further failure, the parents relate to those expectations of failure, rather than to the child's inherent potential for development.

The case study presented here explores some of the above issues in the context of therapeutic work with a depressed mother experiencing relationship difficulties with her multiply disabled infant daughter. At the time of writing this work is still ongoing but already has highlighted a number of themes illustrating the plight of disabled children and the parents who look after them. In this particular case, the life history of the mother has made a particularly significant impact on a situation that would already be difficult and evoke sadness. Each parent has a unique history that will affect the course of the parent–child relationship in a positive or negative way. Some parents will bring the experiences of a reasonably secure attachment relationship with their own parents to the relationship with their child. Others may have parenting experiences that affect self-concept and expectations about relationships in a particularly negative way so that relationships with children are disadvantaged from the beginning. When the child involved has disabilities, the relationship is multiply disadvantaged because past experiences and relationships will resonate with present experiences and relationships. The following case is complex, therefore, because the mother involved had difficult relationships with her parents together with traumatic experiences, contributing to mental health difficulties before her disabled daughter was born.

The referral

Jenny, aged 32, and her daughter, Rebecca, aged 13 months, were referred for counselling and relationship work by a social worker from an adult mental health team. Jenny had attended their postnatal support group because of depression following the birth of her son, Jonathan, three years earlier. She took antidepressant medication and apparently made a good recovery. Jenny started to attend the group again 18 months later when she was expecting her daughter and from late in the pregnancy took antidepressant medication. Rebecca was born three days post term following a normal birth and there were no significant concerns at first. However, by the time she was between five and 12 weeks old, both her eyes were squinting upwards and inwards and Jenny began to worry that something more serious was wrong with her. Two months later results of scans revealed the shocking news that Rebecca's brain had not developed normally and that she would be severely disabled. Furthermore, Jenny experienced additional trauma two months later when she was informed that Rebecca would be partially sighted.

Throughout Rebecca's first year, particularly during the first few months, she was restless, colicky, crying a great deal, and did not feed well. Jenny continued with antidepressant medication for a period until a psychiatrist advised her that it might have interfered with the normal bereavement process associated with having a child with disabilities. However, after stopping the medication, Jenny became highly distressed and said that she could no longer care for Rebecca. This coincided with the period around Rebecca's first birthday, which should have been a time for celebration but served to increase Jenny's pain further. At the time of the referral one month later, Jenny reported having no 'normal' feelings for Rebecca; she did not feel the intense rejection experienced earlier, but stated that she felt nothing. In contrast, although she experienced early difficulties with her son, Jonathan, because of depression, Jenny felt that they had a close and loving relationship. She expressed the desire to conceive another child but felt that first, she should develop an appropriate relationship with Rebecca. Jenny was very self-critical, feeling that she was an unfit mother while she was unable to form a relationship with Rebecca, contributing to her depression and feelings of low self-esteem.

Measurement issues

In the absence of a reliable quantitative measure of mother–infant attachment, progress in the therapy was monitored through self-report from the client and from observations (see mother–infant observation below).

Counselling sessions were reviewed at regular intervals in order to chart progress, summarise issues, renegotiate further blocks of sessions, and agree on the focus of future work. In addition, the client completed anxiety and depression questionnaires (Beck Depression Inventory and Hospital Anxiety and Depression Scale) at regular intervals so that wellbeing could be monitored.

Observations of mother and child

Mother–infant observation in psychodynamically orientated training

Based on her experiences of the usefulness of detailed mother–infant observation in informing clinical work, Esther Bick (1964) initiated the inclusion of this type of observation in psychodynamic psychotherapy training at the Tavistock Clinic, London, in 1948, and it has been adopted by other training institutes since that time. Furthermore, this component of training has been included by the Tavistock in its course on psychodynamic work in learning disability. The observation experience enables the student and therapist to gain a greater understanding of body language, interactions, and the fundamentals of personality development within the context of the child's developing relationship with its parent. Harris (1977, pp. 297–8) noted:

> For most people other than the mother concerned the movements of a small baby are chaotic and fairly meaningless, except in gener-alised behaviour terms. One has to allow oneself to come close to the baby in order to see and retain details, and to cope with the emotional impact and struggle with a great deal of uncertainty in oneself before understandable patterns begin to emerge.

In the context of training, the individual is expected to be a receptive observer only and to learn to refrain from any action. With practice, this experience enables the student to remain in the 'here and now', absorbing the details of the interactions, emotions, and body language of the parent and child observed while priming an awareness of the emotional impact of the scene upon the self. Within therapy, the observation experience can help the therapist to become aware of minute emotional and behavioural indicators that keep him or her in touch with the reality of the client's experiences rather than resorting to premature applications of theory. When these observations and feelings are taken into account, they can add dimension to the quality of later work. In relation to the case presented here, observations of Jenny with her daughter provided valuable insight into the parent–child relationship and aided the counselling process generally.

The first session

Jenny attended for the first assessment session with Rebecca. The squint in both of Rebecca's eyes made her disabilities obvious to the world but, in acknowledging my initial impressions of sadness, I could appreciate some of Jenny's painful feelings about her daughter as well as her experiences of other people's initial curiosity or voyeurism. Brazelton and Cramer (1991, p. 161) pointed out:

> The reaction of disappointment and grief is particularly pronounced if the child carries a visible defect, especially affecting the face (like a cleft lip), or a disease affecting the central nervous system or eyes.

Rebecca was seated on Jenny's knee so that she was sat facing away but close to her mother's body. She moaned and squirmed, pushing her back against Jenny in an apparent attempt to anchor herself as her body, head and limbs moved constantly, seeming to have a mind of their own. I continued to observe Rebecca as Jenny began to describe her experiences and her feelings and imagined a similar struggle within Jenny herself, as she suffered the torment of her thoughts and feelings towards Rebecca. As she spoke, she moved Rebecca into a sequence of positions: on her back; cycling her legs in the air; supporting her on her feet; and sat on the edge of her knee at arm's length. Jenny never seemed comfortable holding Rebecca and appeared to be subconsciously engaged in a never-ending search for a mutually comfortable way to be with her daughter.

Rebecca was noticeably calmer when she could push against her mother's body or when Jenny provided an assortment of teething rings and other hard toys to rub against her gums and to bite on. When I commented on this, Jenny said that movement was also important for Rebecca and she described her contentment over long periods when placed on a vibrating cushion or in a battery-operated swinging chair. I imagined that this was how Rebecca held herself together in the face of the obvious struggle to gain a physiological, cognitive, and emotional equilibrium in the world. Rebecca was not only physically and mentally disabled by her condition but it was obvious also that she could not always depend on what Wilfred Bion described as the container–contained dynamic in the relationship with her grieving mother. In Raphael-Leff's (1993, p. 52) words:

> There is a psychoanalytic idea of a mother as a 'container'. Wilfred Bion proposed that, ideally, mothers, who are the recipients of their baby's anxieties 'contain' these until the infant has established a notion of his or her own inner space in which to keep them. A 'good' mother will hold the baby's unthinkable thoughts, mentally digest them through her 'maternal reverie', and then convey the mitigated emotions so that they can be safely taken back by the infant.

When there is not enough containment, children may have to rely on other means of maintaining a sense of integrity. Miller et al. (1989, pp. 37–8) described Esther Bick's observations:

> Bick felt that some infants came to rely too heavily on an active focusing on, and clinging to the inanimate physical environment as a means of holding their sense of themselves together, rather than depending on human contact. This means of acquiring a sense of identity came to be described as adhesive identification . . . She felt that, in a similar predicament, other children tried to develop feelings of being whole largely through using their experience of their own muscular tensions or the experience of motion . . . Bick called this a second skin formation. Such a 'skin' is not conducive to the development of a mental experience of a skin/container that can both hold together a sense of identity and yet remain permeable to emotional experience.

During later sessions with Jenny she was to describe a reluctance to disturb Rebecca if she was content in her chair swing swiping at her toys, fearing her wrath about being taken away from the rhythmic rocking and familiar playthings. Jenny found the experience of Rebecca's distress too overwhelming, bringing feelings of guilt, anger and helplessness. She often felt unable to hold Rebecca until she had calmed down, resorting to the swinging chair or vibrating cushion to re-establish calm and contentment in her daughter. Jenny described later that she felt that Rebecca's distress increased when she held her daughter and that she seemed to want to push her mother away but was unable to do so.

Jenny described guilty feelings about Rebecca's condition and said that she felt responsible. Her eyes filled with tears, her body was tense, and she moved Rebecca to the edge of her knee, supporting her back with her hand. Rebecca, suddenly deprived of the more secure anchorage of her mother's body, began to moan fretfully and her arms and legs flailed chaotically. I observed similar fretting again when Jenny began to weep about the constant physical and emotional drain of caring for Rebecca, and her particular sadness because Rebecca was unable to see, increasing the feeling of being cut-off from one another. Rebecca seemed to be experiencing her mother's distress through her tension and body language so I commented about this to Jenny, saying that Rebecca appeared to be 'tuning in' to her mother's sadness and distress, becoming distressed herself. Sinason (1992) distinguished between cognitive and emotional intelligence, pointing out that it is possible for an individual to be emotionally sensitive and perceptive despite limited cognitive abilities. Jenny had not noticed how she could affect Rebecca's emotional wellbeing before but said that it made sense because whenever she visited her mother, with whom she had a very difficult relationship, Jenny was always tense and Rebecca seemed to 'scream for most of the time'. Differentiating between emotional and cognitive functioning seemed to increase Jenny's optimism about their relationship in the future.

Observation of Jenny playing with Rebecca

In addition to a counselling approach, part of the intended work with Jenny and Rebecca was to bring them together in play through what Daniel Stern (1985) described as 'attunement'. Since young infants have to learn to regulate various physiological systems before they can pay full attention to outside stimuli, initially a mother has to be able to adapt to the child's need to switch attention on and off. When a physiological homeostasis begins to develop, the mother can begin to woo her child into a repertoire of mirroring games that are sensitive to intensity, rhythm, form and duration. As such, she treats all responses as intentional and gives them meaning. Gradually, autonomy emerges in the infant and the mother must learn to recognise and encourage child-led searches for, and responses to, social and environmental stimuli. This process is somewhat protracted in children struggling with multiple disabilities, making attunement much more difficult for mother and child. In addition, maternal depression is one of the most common causes of failure in attunement between parent and infant (Brazelton and Cramer 1991).

Interventions with parents in order to facilitate attunement and attachment have involved highlighting the child's individual characteristics; modelling and supporting interactions with a disabled child (Als 1982); modelling and supporting interactions in conjunction with individual psychotherapy (Watanabe 1994); and structured play approaches in conjunction with group therapy (Binney et al. 1994). Brazelton and Cramer (1991, p. 214) pointed out:

> Whatever technique is used (guidance, support, psychotherapy), the clinician should be very attentive to the problem of self-esteem. Attachment . . . can develop only if parents can resolve the wound to their self-image. This often requires special help. One should never forget that a baby begins inside the mother. As such, a newborn represents in a visible way the innermost part of herself.

The following account is a description of an initial observation of Jenny playing with Rebecca during an early play session and illustrates some of the difficulties encountered in the relationship.

Rebecca was in the swinging chair on my arrival. She was very sleepy but her body and limbs were writhing and seemed to be depriving her of the rest she was seeking. Rebecca was still for about 15 seconds, seeming to have drifted into sleep, then her body jerked into movement again, dragging her back to the surface. She started to fret and her body and limbs thrashed around more energetically for a while. Gradually, she became still again and she seemed to be at peace, only to be disturbed again by her own movements. When I commented to Jenny about Rebecca's struggle, she said that she had been held more than usual during the family's holiday away from home the previous week, and this was what she wanted. We observed Rebecca's movements and fretting together in silence for a few moments but Jenny could no longer bear to hear her daughter's distress. She removed Rebecca from the chair and placed her on a sheepskin rug saying that sometimes Rebecca could relax to sleep on this soft bed. Rebecca's arms and legs thrashed in the air and her crying increased in intensity. Jenny chided her but after a few seconds, unable to bear hearing her daughter's distress any longer, she picked her up and rocked her in her arms. Rebecca was calm immediately. It appeared that Rebecca's experiences of being held frequently the week before, particularly by her father, had stimulated a desire to be held in this way again.

I had talked to Jenny about the play approach intended and provided some written information about child-centred, empathic approaches to encouraging interactions with children with disabilities (Prevezer 1991). Such an approach initially would involve responding to the spontaneous sounds and movements of the child as if they are intentionally communicative. Gradually, the child may be encouraged to start using them intentionally, will learn to anticipate, and eventually will begin to initiate interactions. As I began to review this approach with Jenny she began to cast doubt on Rebecca's ability to communicate and play. She described how Rebecca did not seem to respond to overtures from the people around her and although she could smile this was not social smiling and appeared to be random. For example, she could be sitting in her chair smiling at nothing in particular. Jenny went on to say that Rebecca's responses were the same with everyone and she did not seem to differentiate between them. Indeed, she did not feel more special to Rebecca than any other person.

I felt overwhelmed by Jenny's negativity about her daughter for a few moments, feeling the hopelessness she had projected into me. I watched Rebecca as she sat leaning against her mother's body facing outwards. A toy had been placed between her uncoordinated hands and I could see that she was struggling to take it to her mouth to explore. I commented on this attempt to Jenny and observed at the same time that Rebecca was trying to look at me as I spoke. She turned her head to one side and seemed to be trying to focus by looking sideways. I smiled at her but she did not respond. However, after being put onto her back by Jenny, I was struck by how she thrust her head back to watch me and how her eyes tracked my movements as I approached her. During previous visits, I had observed that Rebecca could swipe at toys intentionally and repeatedly when placed in front of her. She responded to noisy toys and seemed to derive much pleasure from swiping at playthings until they were knocked off her tray onto the floor. Indeed, she had learned that she could impact on her world with some predictability. As I remembered this evidence of Rebecca's development together with the present scene, the hopelessness dissipated.

I asked Jenny if she would be able to play with Rebecca in my presence and although she felt nervous, agreed to do so. Jenny opted to play singing-action games such as 'Pat-a-cake', 'Round-and-round the garden', and 'Wind the bobbin'. Rebecca showed obvious enjoyment through smiles and when Jenny played 'Wind the bobbin' moving her legs, Rebecca giggled delightfully. Rebecca enjoyed also being pulled up onto her feet while Jenny repeated 'up-up-up . . .' in a rising intonation. Afterwards, I told Jenny that she had played with Rebecca beautifully. It was notable that she gave Rebecca a number of kisses and blew raspberries against her forehead. We were both filled with optimism and it was agreed that Jenny would make some time to play with Rebecca like this each day. Jenny commented at this point that she felt they had missed out on the normal play for pleasure between mother and child because 'play' always involved working towards goals (as in portage or physiotherapy).

Unfortunately, the optimism was short-lived as on the next visit one week later, Jenny was depressed. Rebecca was reported to be unwell and difficult when awake and she had been reluctant to disturb Rebecca when she was peaceful and settled, fearful of precipitating further distress. Jenny reported that she had observed often that Rebecca did not like to experience a sudden change in position. For example, during physiotherapy exercises, she would start to cry when she was laid down in a prone position unless 'tricked' by the physiotherapist moving her very slowly. Jenny felt, therefore, that the sudden change in position when she was picked up disturbed Rebecca too much and caused distress. During a later session, however, Jenny disclosed that she had to some extent avoided playing with Rebecca because she found it too painful to have emotional contact with her. Subsequent sessions involved the exploration of the kinds of feelings evoked in Jenny when she engaged emotionally with her daughter.

Emerging themes during counselling

Expectations of loss and failure of attachment

Jenny described how she did not feel anything for Rebecca and said that it was like looking after another person's child. Although she felt able to care for her daughter's physical needs, the lack of emotional bonding created the feeling that eventually she would be handing Rebecca over to someone else as she had done in her former occupation as a nanny. Jenny indicated that she had a good knowledge about Rebecca's condition and that she had been given an honest prognosis by the paediatrician involved. She added that in the early months after Rebecca's disabilities were diagnosed, she believed and hoped that Rebecca would die, and in order to protect herself, held back from developing a relationship. McFadyen (1994) in her book about special care babies and their developing relationships commented that a combination of expectations about loss, doubts about being able to care for the child, feelings of being peripheral because of the many professionals involved, and the child's physical appearance, all contribute to a mother's difficulties in 'owning' her child. Since Rebecca had survived, Jenny felt that she should establish a relationship with her for both their sakes, especially as she was planning to conceive another child.

Bereavement issues

In relation to having a child with disabilities, it is argued that the bereavement response is about loss of the idealised pre-birth fantasy child who is imbued with intelligence and other characteristics associated with the hopes and desires of the parents (Brazelton and Cramer 1991; Raphael-Leff 1993; Bungener and McCormack 1994). Confronted with a child with disabilities, parents may move through a number of phases involving shock, panic, denial, grief, guilt, anger, bargaining (conditional acceptance) and acceptance (Bicknell 1983; Hall 1984). The process is likely to involve the re-experiencing of loss at significant stages such as when the child does not reach milestones at the same rate as other children and at critical periods in the life cycle of the family (Ditchfield 1992; Hall 1984).

For Jenny, the loss of her idealised imaginary child was still a source of extreme emotional pain and despair. She had experienced the shock of diagnosis during Rebecca's early months and, to some extent, still moved in and out of panic and denial about her ability to care for Rebecca and accept the reality of her condition. Jenny's home was crammed with toys and equipment from all over the country devised for children with special needs, in a quest to stimulate and please her daughter and reduce the impact of her disabilities as much as possible. She consulted also a number of medical professionals in order to establish whether pharmacological or surgical procedures could improve Rebecca's functioning. Guilt was a particular issue for Jenny as she believed that somehow she must have damaged the foetus. Maybe, she questioned, it was something she had ingested at a critical time, perhaps she had exposed herself to something toxic, or maybe she had hurt the foetus through some physical activity. She had been informed that there was no genetic link and found it difficult to believe that chance factors beyond her control could be responsible. At a later stage in the counselling process, Jenny reported that during her pregnancy, she felt resentful at times towards the developing baby inside her and sometimes felt that she did not want to have this child. On discovering that Rebecca had severe disabilities, she felt that somehow her thoughts and feelings had damaged her child or that she was being punished for having them. Alternatively, she wondered whether the negative feelings about the new baby during pregnancy were a warning sign that all was not well and that she should have alerted the medical professionals at the time. Increasing her sense of responsibility, Jenny's mother had been critical about her desire to have a second child, commenting insensitively that, like herself, she should have been satisfied with one and she only had herself to blame. Jenny had not yet reached the stages of bargaining or acceptance but moved in and out of grieving in conjunction with alternating periods of emotional numbness and emotional crises arising from the strain of caring for Rebecca. The pain of having a daughter with multiple disabilities was also renewed regularly when Jenny met with other mothers and saw children of a similar age to Rebecca reaching their developmental milestones.

Jenny was determined to have another child because she wanted Jonathan to have the benefit of a normal sibling relationship, something she felt Rebecca could not provide. She had hated being an only child herself because she had felt isolated and lonely. Although it was intended that Jenny would be working on her relationship with Rebecca before conceiving another child, shortly after the beginning of therapy, Jenny announced that she was pregnant again. Later investigations revealed that she was having another daughter. During the early stages of pregnancy when she had extensive tests to check the status of the foetus, Jenny aired fears about her new baby being disabled in some way. If the tests revealed some abnormality, would she have an abortion? If she had an abortion, how would this make her feel about Rebecca? There were no easy answers and the prospect of having to make such choices was depressing. Eventually, when the tests and scans indicated that the baby appeared to be growing normally, Jenny moved on to talk about her fear and guilt that the new daughter would replace Rebecca in her affections, and the fantasy child she did not have would be born. Jenny had begun the process of redecorating the nursery for the new baby and Rebecca had been moved out to another bedroom. She did not see it primarily as preparation for her new daughter, however, but as an attempt to exorcise the painful memories associated with the arrival of Rebecca. This time, she wanted to 'get it right' and the new decorations in the nursery were like 'wiping the slate clean' again.

Ghosts from the past

During the course of the sessions, Jenny talked about experiences from her past. She described a lonely, unhappy childhood with an emotionally distant, controlling mother and a father who was often absent because he travelled extensively on business. When her father was at home, Jenny enjoyed some emotional nurturing but at the cost of being sexually abused between the ages of about seven and nine years of age. Jenny's early memories were vague and generalised but she recalled a mother who could not understand why her daughter did not conform to book descriptions of child rearing, and would punish messiness or behaviour that was not perfect. Emotions such as anger and distress could not be contained by her mother and Jenny learned to put them away. During her late teenage years Jenny was raped and, in her twenties, she was afflicted by anorexia nervosa. Although she had received therapy in order to resolve the issues involved some years earlier, becoming a mother of a disabled child had rekindled some of the emotional pain.

In relation to Jenny's present experiences of Rebecca, the internalised critical mother was ever present, telling her that she was not good enough. As a result, Jenny would swing from perfectionism on the one hand, in her efforts to care for Rebecca (physical care, carrying out portage and physiotherapy exercises, pacifying distress before it escalated), to being emotionally drained on the other (withdrawing and ignoring her daughter's demands and distress) and in the process feeling angry and a failure. This, in turn, would increase feelings of guilt and she would redouble her efforts again. Furthermore, whenever Jenny went out with Rebecca, she imagined that people thought she was a failure as a mother, seeing her as damaging as well as damaged and inadequate herself. Moreover, Jenny's mother continued to be emotionally abusive and rejecting in the present. She would not refer to Rebecca by name, calling her 'the other one', and when Rebecca was asleep, would suggest that she should be put in another room out of sight and mind. Furthermore, Jenny's mother could not understand why this child was not sent away to be fostered or adopted and would raise the subject repeatedly during visits. Through projective identification, it felt to Jenny that her vulnerable child self was being rejected all over again.

Jenny's experiences of emotional and sexual abuse as a child and being raped as a young adult had deeply damaged her self-image. As such, whenever she regarded her daughter, Rebecca reminded Jenny of how damaged she felt inside. Jenny felt responsible and ashamed of her experiences of abuse and had difficulty in accepting that her natural trust and need for affection as a child had been distorted and abused within the power imbalance of a parent–child relationship. It has to be acknowledged, however, that although abusive, the relationship between Jenny and her father was probably the best source of comfort and love available to her at the time. Such relationships are often the source of great internal conflict and pain when the abused person reviews his or her experiences in later years.

Jenny's vulnerable, internal child was stirred also by distressing thoughts about Rebecca's vulnerability to abuse in the future. Recently, she had watched a news report about a residential home where multiply disabled children had been maltreated by staff and she remembered other past reports of children being sexually abused by adults whilst in their care. Indeed, as Sinason (1993a) pointed out, although estimates of the prevalence of abuse in the learning disabled population vary, it is clear that because of an inherent vulnerability (greater dependency, less able to protect themselves, less able to disclose and so forth), the prevalence rate is likely to be just as high as, if not higher, than in the general population.

Dilemmas

Rebecca's struggle to coordinate and support herself meant that she needed physiotherapy input if she was to make any progress. This would have a payoff for Jenny as well as for Rebecca, as it would increase her independence at a basic level. Unfortunately, however, when taken away from the security of her chair or her mother's lap, in order to be rolled over on the floor and so forth, she became highly distressed. The physiotherapists were highly sensitive to the distress that this caused for Jenny and did not push her to work with Rebecca beyond what was bearable. Jenny was torn between wanting to push Rebecca to her limits in order to reduce her disabilities as much as possible on the one hand, and feeling cruel, heartless and abusive on the other. She would persist on some days and go through the recommended exercises with Rebecca at home. On other days, she could not bear to hear Rebecca's crying and did not persist at all. Indeed, Jenny remarked that when she tried to do the exercises with her daughter she remained upset and unsettled for long periods afterwards, making her reluctant to attempt the exercises with Rebecca in the first place. These experiences also brought her face to face with Rebecca's disabilities and provoked deep, raw, emotional sadness and despair in Jenny. Sinason (1993b) acknowledged the dilemma of care in the context of parents who found it difficult to steer a middle course, resulting in much resentment and distress in the child on the one hand, and lack of development and opportunities missed, on the other. In addition, Jenny's past experiences as a child were having an impact, leading to projective identification. In particular, she talked about how her experiences of being abused as a child had made her sensitive to forcing both her children to do anything they found unpleasant. She did not like to apply Jonathan's eczema cream because it would sting him and make him cry but she knew that it would make things better so she would persist. However, she was uncertain as to whether physiotherapy would have a significant impact on Rebecca's disabilities and whether it was worth the effort and distress. Unfortunately, the professionals involved could not provide her with definite answers in this respect.

One of the aspects of Rebecca's disabilities was the impairment to her vision. In her search for possible medical interventions in this respect, Jenny had been told that surgery was possible but the outcome would be cosmetic. She was faced with the dilemma, therefore, as to whether she should put her daughter through the trauma of hospital admission and surgery. She wondered if this was for Rebecca's sake or for her own.

Progress in the mother–infant relationship

As counselling progressed during the pregnancy, Jenny's mood improved generally and she felt more able to resume efforts to work on her relationship with Rebecca through regular play. During part of our weekly session, she spent time with Rebecca on her lap, playing action-song games with her, talking to her, and holding her close. The play periods were brief and the restlessness observed during the first encounter was still apparent. Nevertheless, Rebecca showed great pleasure through smiles and giggling during these interactions and Jenny was obviously pleased when Rebecca responded in this way. As I observed Rebecca's face, she moved constantly and it was difficult to focus at close quarters on any of her features without feeling slightly dizzy and visually fatigued. I reflected this back to Jenny because in the light of this experience, I could appreciate that efforts to make an emotional link with Rebecca were frustrated by the difficulty in maintaining a visual focus while the movement itself served as a constant reminder of the extent of Rebecca's disabilities. For Rebecca herself, the difficulties of maintaining a physiological, cognitive and emotional equilibrium during her development to this point must have been considerable given the nature of her disabilities. She was, however, able to enjoy the play initiated by her mother but it was notable that she needed to avert her attention to internal physiological and motoric control at regular intervals or, alternatively, she would start to cry. Jenny was highly self-critical so it was important for her to know that the some of the difficulties were related to these factors. Als (1991) noted during observations of mother–infant interactions that a child's development is characterised by phases of temporary disorganisation before new organisation and a period of consolidation can occur. In infants struggling with multiple disabilities, the process was observed to be slow and painful so that, in interactions, the mother's expectation for failure accumulates and she tires of the very wearing demands of attempting to fuel and expand her infant's capabilities. In such circumstances, support for the mother is important so that she can appreciate that when her child moves from averting to full orientation and then to insulated crying, it is a normal and inevitable process in the unfolding of behavioural organisation.

There were some extended periods (three or four days) when Rebecca seemed to be in distress for most of the time. Jenny found these episodes very stressful and tiring because whatever she tried to do to pacify her did not seem to ameliorate Rebecca's distress at all. She took comfort from the fact that Rebecca's behaviour did not change when she was with the respite carer (who related to Rebecca in a very positive and caring way) as this indicated to Jenny that it was not caused by something personal to their relationship or her style of care. She worried, however, that Rebecca was in pain or discomfort and consulted the family's GP and the paediatrician on a number of occasions. Rebecca's crying and screaming provoked a raw emotional pain within Jenny, driving her to persist in consulting medical professionals. Antibiotics and other kinds of medication were prescribed despite the absence of the usual physical symptoms and, on one occasion, she was admitted to the local children's hospital in order to investigate for reflux but no explanation for Rebecca's distress could be found. Jenny was left with the feeling that no one could do anything about Rebecca's difficulties. It was noted, however, that after each of these episodes, Rebecca emerged with new skills and an improved ability to engage and interact for longer periods. Brazelton (1992, p. 168) observed that for premature infants, development proceeds in the protracted manner noted earlier in multiply disabled children but noted further that the periods of reorganisation are interspersed with horrendous periods of disorganisation. He commented:

> For example, just before he sits up or crawls or stands or walks, a premature infant can be expected to fall apart. He will cry more unpredictably and will be harder to comfort; he will start waking up at night all over again; he will cry whenever one turns one's back; he will act as if nothing can really satisfy him. Unless his parents can learn that this precedes another spurt in development and thereby gain courage, they, too, will fall apart. And each will drag down the other.

Jenny could accept this information at one level but she had observed that the antibiotic treatment seemed to work and was, therefore, not entirely convinced that such distress could be a natural part of Rebecca's development. It was suggested to her that the process of consulting a medical professional had helped to contain her own distress and anxieties which, in turn, had helped to restore an emotional equilibrium within Rebecca. Whatever the explanation for Rebecca's apparent recovery might be, the degree of distress evoked within Jenny led her to seek medication for Rebecca each time these episodes occurred.

A particular issue for Jenny was the extent of Rebecca's dependency on herself and others. Jenny had learnt from early childhood that being dependent could provoke extremely negative responses from her own mother and in response, therefore, she learnt to submerge her attachment needs (Bowlby 1969), becoming independent physically and emotionally from an early age. The internalised critical mother within Jenny resented Rebecca for her constant demands and extensive dependence whereas the needy, dependent child part of herself who had not received adequate love and containment was projected into Rebecca. Having a daughter with disabilities rather than a son also meant that Jenny could see parts of herself more easily in Rebecca. Rebecca's cries and her general dependency were a constant source of pain, therefore, whenever Jenny made emotional contact with her daughter during the play sessions. Although it was agreed that Jenny would spend some time each day playing with Rebecca, in practice Jenny could not do this without support within our sessions. In between sessions, there were always obstacles to working on the relationship; Rebecca was unwell, there was not enough time, Jenny felt too exhausted, or she felt too depressed. As the birth of Jenny's second daughter approached, she found it increasingly more difficult to physically accommodate

Rebecca on her lap. Nevertheless, Jenny was encouraged to play with Rebecca lying on the floor or seated in a chair.

A new daughter

Jenny's second daughter, Leah, was born without any complications and appeared to be well and functioning normally. However, the experience of her new daughter was marred initially by worries that she would start to develop problems. Gradually, Jenny started to show signs of post-natal depression and found the experience of caring for all three children very difficult. She reported feeling detached from Leah and experienced her birth and subsequent development as a reminder of the early months with Rebecca. Jenny said that she was frightened of developing a close bond with Leah because she was afraid that the same things would happen again. The sessions at this time were spent examining Jenny's fears in the context of her past traumatic experiences with Rebecca. Rebecca's disabilities were not confirmed until she was around five months old, although suspicions that something was wrong arose well before that time. Leah, however, was very different from her sister during the early stages of development, being a notably alert child, constantly monitoring her mother and the environment generally. Emphasising the differences between them helped Jenny to regain some perspective but her mood remained quite low.

Jenny's husband, Peter, encouraged her to take antidepressant medication but Jenny resisted because she wanted to breast-feed Leah. This caused a fair amount of conflict in their relationship because Peter had agreed to a third child on the basis that Jenny had said she would be able to cope. He felt that refusing to take medication was irresponsible and he was resentful because she was not coping as she said she would. As a result, Jenny felt that she could not turn to him for support and felt increasingly angry and isolated. She reached crisis-point during a two-week break in therapy (annual leave) and went to visit her GP who prescribed antidepressant medication. Shortly afterwards, her mood began to improve. It was notable that this crisis coincided with Jenny's last crisis one year previously (immediately after Rebecca's birthday), when she reported that she was no longer able to care for Rebecca.

Work with Jenny and Rebecca over the following months was disrupted by Jenny having to go into hospital for major surgery. Social services provided Jenny with extra childcare support within the home and through extra respite care, making it difficult for me to see Jenny on her own with Rebecca. When a visit was possible, however, the time was spent encouraging the relationship play work with Rebecca begun prior to the birth of Leah. Leah was always present, so Jenny was encouraged to work in this way with both children. While Jenny played with Rebecca, I would model interactions and play with Leah. The process was repeated when the children were swapped over. Jenny continued to need support in order to do this work, however, as the same obstacles to continuing the work between sessions were reiterated.

As the childcare support fell away because Jenny had recovered physically, she started to report depressed feelings again. This time she had thoughts of killing herself. It was noted that during pregnancy and when in the sick role, Jenny did not have to think about taking care of the needs of others or take on her usual competent person role to the same extent. However, when the childcare support was reduced, this meant that, in particular, Jenny had to spend more time with Rebecca, tending to her needs. When Jenny was encouraged to reflect on her situation, she began to talk about wanting to reject Rebecca but believed that she could not do anything about it and felt trapped. On the one hand, she felt guilty and ashamed that she felt this way, believing that she was a failure as a mother, and on the other she knew that Peter had developed a bond with Rebecca and would be devastated to lose her. At the same time, she felt frustrated with Peter because he was unable to understand why Jenny could not pull herself out of the depression by focusing on the positive aspects of Rebecca. They had stopped communicating in this respect and Jenny felt helpless, hopeless, and alone; a situation that resonated strongly with her experiences as a child. In particular, she felt trapped by her obligations to look after Rebecca, much as she had felt trapped by the abusive relationship with her father.

Although Jenny had reached the depths of despair, facing her true feelings about Rebecca in the context of supportive counselling helped her to gain a perspective and move on to a new phase in therapy. In particular, she agreed to include Peter in a joint session so that communication between them could be facilitated. This had been suggested on a number of previous occasions but Jenny had felt that Peter would not understand and would be reluctant to attend. Hall (1984) pointed out that parents' responses to having a child with disabilities can differ and this can be a potential source of conflict and disharmony, often resulting in relationships collapsing under the strain. Furthermore, these differences and opinions can be exacerbated if the parents are not seen and counselled together. At the time of writing, Peter had agreed to attend for one session that seemed to be a fruitful experience for both parties. During this session, Peter was able to talk for the first time to Jenny about some of the sad feelings he had for Rebecca. His coping response was to try to look at all the positives and this strategy had helped him to develop a good relationship with his disabled daughter who he could see was a little person with her own personality. Peter acknowledged further that he had positive experiences of being parented, which made it easier to develop good relationships with his children. Jenny said that she felt relieved to hear that Peter had some of the same sad feelings as herself, often feeling criticised and isolated because he never talked about his internal sadness, emphasising instead that she should look on the positive side. Perhaps Peter was afraid that Jenny would be engulfed by her sad feelings or she would openly reject Rebecca if he acknowledged how she felt. By the end of the session, Peter and Jenny had agreed that they would try to communicate their true feelings to one another about Rebecca and acknowledge the painful times together. If they could manage to communicate in this way, it was felt that Jenny could benefit from much-needed emotional support that, in turn, might enable her to regain a perspective on life and share Peter's positive attitude towards Rebecca.

Ethical issues

In the course of writing about a clinical case in such detail, I became troubled by the ethical implications of telling someone's story without obtaining consent to do so. I consulted a number of colleagues about this dilemma, discussing the advantages and disadvantages of sharing this information with the client and obtained a number of different opinions. One colleague felt that there was no need to involve the client if identifying information was changed. Another colleague was concerned that sharing information about the counselling process could be damaging to a client but felt that, without informed consent, such a piece could not be published. An American colleague felt that whilst care should be taken to avoid damaging the client and the therapist–client relationship, clients should also be given credit for their ability to survive adversity and respected for their strengths when making such ethical decisions. An alternative suggestion given by another colleague was to write about a number of cases in less detail so that ethical permission did not need to be sought. Unfortunately this latter suggestion would have defeated the object of the present book which aims to focus on the process of working with a particular individual within the particular models and approaches of each author, rather than using case examples to support particular models and theories.

In the end, because of the range of opinions expressed, it was felt that I would need to use my own clinical and ethical judgement in this case to determine what to do. I decided to approach the client for her permission to submit the case for publication based on the considerable courage and strength she had shown in facing the many painful issues raised during the counselling process. The client was very positive about her story being told within the context of the present book and said that she would like to read the manuscript. It was agreed that the manuscript could be used to compare perspectives as well as being a useful basis for future therapy.

When she had read the manuscript, the client reported that the detailed observations, in particular, had helped her to appreciate the situation from her daughter's perspective for the first time, evoking feelings of sadness on her behalf. The client felt that the story told was an accurate account of the feelings and dilemmas experienced but asked for some extra information to be included where she felt that it did not tell the full story. This information has been incorporated into the main body of the present chapter. It should be noted further that all identifying information about the case has been changed in order to protect the client and her family.

Summary

The above case study involves a number of themes and issues in relation to the experience of being the parent of a child with severe learning disabilities. These are presented in the context of a complex case involving a mother with a difficult life history, which has made its own particular impact on a situation that would already evoke much sadness. The strength and courage shown by this mother to face the many painful issues highlighted during counselling has been considerable.

In this case, the mother had not formed a close relationship with her multiply-disabled infant, hoping that she would not survive so that she would not have to make painful emotional connections with her daughter. The death wish was part of a spectrum of ambivalent feelings, however, of which guilt and empathy were a part. The guilty feelings from an internalised critical mother pushed this woman to work in therapy in order to resolve the relationship with her daughter and the empathic feelings came from her past experiences of being rejected and abused as a child. At the same time, the resonance between the damaged inner child of the mother and the presence of her disabled daughter caused extreme emotional turmoil and pain; the daughter acting as a mirror to the damage she felt inside. She learnt to switch off from her daughter in order to protect herself from the distress but in the process could not always act as a reliable container or encourage interaction. The infant managed to survive but was highly dependent on the physical environment for holding herself together, partly because of the nature of her disability that threatened her physiological and psychological integrity. The fact that her daughter could survive and derive enjoyment from non-human forms of contact promoted the belief in the mother that she did not have any impact on her little girl as she did not appear to respond to her in any special way. In the meantime, however, this little girl apparently enjoyed a good relationship with her father and the respite carer, providing a basis for encouraging development and interaction.

When the mother did connect with her daughter, she was confronted with the loss of her perfect fantasy child. The grief and shame felt was increased at frequent intervals by perceived reactions and curiosity whenever she took her daughter out. Both inside and outside her home, she was faced also with children who were reaching several developmental milestones she knew her daughter had not achieved. Furthermore, although her efforts to obtain material aids and medical input in order to reduce the disabilities was heroic, she was always confronted in the end with the reality that the disabilities would remain. There were also dilemmas regarding the treatments that Rebecca should or could have in order to reduce her disabilities or to make her look more acceptable.

Throughout the pregnancy with her second daughter, this mother became worried that she would reject her disabled child and the new daughter would become the perfect fantasy child that her first daughter could never be. After the birth of their second daughter, the parents' relationship became strained and distant, leaving the mother feeling isolated, resentful, and trapped. This situation resonated strongly with her childhood experiences and fuelled the rejection felt towards her disabled daughter who continued to be demanding and, at times, difficult to pacify because of her development. Eventually, she began to have suicidal thoughts because it seemed to be the only way out. With supportive counselling which acknowledged the extent of her guilty and rejecting feelings, the mother agreed to the inclusion of her partner in one of the sessions.

At the time of writing, the session had taken place and this initial contact indicated that there was sufficient strength in their relationship to work on communication and mutual support issues.

Conclusions

In the course of writing up a case for publication it would have been gratifying to end the present paper with an account of a satisfactory resolution to this piece of clinical work. However, it is likely, given the complexity of the issues, that the clinical work with this particular family will continue for some time yet. Irrespective of the complexity of a particular case, it should be noted that parents of children with severe disabilities will continue to have moments of sadness, guilt, anger or anxiety throughout their lives as life events (such as deaths, divorce, redundancy) and lifespan issues (such as developmental milestones, respite care, school, care during adulthood) make their impact. Sometimes, parents and their children have crises at these times and need to return for professional help or seek support until the particular problems have been resolved. As such, the work relating to having a son or daughter with a disability is a lifelong process.

Chapter 7
James: counselling an adult with articulation problems

DIANA SYDER

A personal journey – the case study – major themes that emerged in the first three months – therapy, progress and change – evaluation – writing up – articulation therapy with adults: transfer and maintenance – implications for children with 'minor' articulatory disorders.

A personal journey

During my first five years as a speech and language therapist, the job seemed to require me to know more about the condition of being human than anything else. I was working on a neurosurgical ward and all the big life questions seemed to crop up over and over again. Even at 27 I had barely started to sort out these questions for myself and certainly didn't feel skilled enough to help others do the same. Knowing more facts did not help. I could not escape the suspicion that I was being paid to be a 'nice lady'. A nurse who attended a workshop I had just led, told me afterwards at the bus stop that she expected the patients would feel better just by talking to me. At the time I felt affronted, now I realise this was one of the biggest compliments she could have paid me. Not long after this I attended a co-counselling course and went on a weekend workshop dealing with loss. It was an opening into a different world. A little later, events in my personal life finally steered me into my own counselling. During a two-year period of therapy I read voraciously, admittedly motivated by my own needs, but nevertheless what I learned and experienced spilled into my own work situation and gave me a whole new set of skills, attitudes, awarenesses and understandings. The nice lady had gone.

From then on I attended whatever short courses I could manage: focused expressive therapy, one term of psychodrama, Gestalt, interpersonal process recall (IPR) and assorted others. I was also beginning to raise issues of counselling and supervision within my service. I attended a large one-day conference on supervision and was the only speech and language therapist there. A few years later I entered therapy again and this time chose to work with a Gestalt therapist.

Thus I arrive at my present position with a varied background made up of hands-on experience and a wide-ranging though patchy theoretical knowledge. In this I am like the majority of speech and language therapists who have picked up skills and knowledge from a variety of sources over the years and am therefore, perhaps more than the other authors, representative of the position of most speech and language therapists.

I have found it helpful to stop and consider what ideas, from which models, do inform my work. Carl Rogers' words (1967) come immediately into my head

> Gradually my experience has forced me to conclude that the individual has within himself the capacity and the tendency, latent if not evident, to move forward toward maturity. In a suitable psychological climate this tendency is released and becomes actual rather than potential.

In my work with James I believed that he had the potential to move and change, to become someone he likes and to achieve enough of his dreams to enjoy life. Again to quote from Rogers (1967), I expected James to move

> . . . toward a conception of himself as a person of worth, as a self-directing person, able to form his standards and values upon the basis of his own experience . . . The initial discrepancy between the self that he is and the self he wants to be is greatly diminished.

Rogers (1967) extrapolates to say that the client 'actually comes to like himself. This is not a bragging or self-assertive liking; it is rather a quiet pleasure in being one's self.' So throughout our work together I tried to trust James' ability to find his own route through, doing my best to reject the role of expert that he offered me and in fact pressured me to take. In keeping with such a model we had an open-ended contract regarding the length of therapy, trusting we would both recognise when the time was right to finish.

I also believe the relationship between therapist and client is crucial. So for someone like James, who had never risked such an intimate relationship before, it was important to hold the boundaries of this relationship and allow it to be used as a starting point for reconsidering other relationships in his life. Thus while some of our work operated at a cognitive level, challenging and offering alternatives to James's thought patterns, we also worked at a feeling level and paid attention to what was happening in the here and now between us. In addition I believe that the way we relate to people as adults is influenced by our early family relationships and therefore saw it as important to explore how James operated within his family when he was young, especially as he traced the beginning of his difficulties back to when he was eight years old.

The case study

Therapy prior to referral

At the point of referral in May 1995, James had undergone several months of electropalatography (EPG) therapy for intransigent lateralisation of sibilant fricatives and affricates and as a result had modified fricatives and affricates within the clinic. He was still dependent on feedback from the computer and was reluctant to use a tape recorder for self-monitoring. At this point, my colleague, Sara Howard, was unclear about the best way of helping James transfer his fledgeling skills outside the clinic and although we talked in behavioural terms, she did tell me James was shy and withdrawn and that she felt he would benefit from more generic counselling.

Biographical details

James was in his late twenties, in full-time professional employment and had extended contact with the public. He lived in his own house. His father had died 13 years earlier. His mother was still living and he saw her regularly. There were twin sisters, older than James but they lived away and James had no contact with them. There were no other speech problems in the family and James' speech had never been openly discussed. James was teased at school but remembered being confident until his teens. He reported being close to his father and remembers him trying to help correct his speech when he was young. He expressed irritation with his mother who he experienced as overcritical, manipulative and denigratory, although he had strong loyalties to her. There was no contact between James and either of the twins, who did not have much contact either with each other, or their mother. He had had ear infections in childhood with surgery at about six years. Otherwise no medical history of note.

Initial assessment

In telling me about himself, James placed much emphasis on speech and correct pronunciation but demonstrated little awareness of other aspects of communication. He talked about avoiding situations, described himself as shy and made the link between this and his speech. He referred repeatedly to 'the goal' and though he couldn't tell me exactly what the goal was, it was framed in terms of 'new /s/' versus 'old /s/'. James felt that if his speech changed, everything else would automatically fall into place, but again at this stage, although I got no clear sense of what 'everything else' was, I did begin to form the impression that even if James' articulation were transformed, it wouldn't bring about the radical change in his circumstances that he wanted.

James reported that speech worsened:

- in spontaneous conversation;
- when speaking quickly;
- in long sentences.

He spoke of being respected because of his authority in his job. I noticed a change in his demeanour when at one point I began to talk about elements of our personalities that we don't allow ourselves to express and he looked alert and showed interest in this idea. In general conversation James' fricatives were still noticeably disordered, otherwise he presented as a pleasant and intelligent young man and appeared to be well motivated. He was somewhat concrete in his description of and approach to his problems and needed considerable help to elaborate. I was aware of having to work hard to facilitate our conversation and not being altogether successful in avoiding a question/answer format. We agreed to meet for eight one-hour sessions in the first instance and that EPG practice with Sara would continue independently during this time. After eight weeks we would review.

Rationale of therapy

Difficult. When Sara and I first talked, our initial thoughts had been that I would work on a behavioural generalisation programme, given that James had already acquired a set of new articulatory skills and modified his behaviour in a clinic context. Personal construct theory (PCT) provided me with a useful concept for organising James' problems. 'When clients mention that their speech is not as it should be our first task is to determine at what level change should be effected' (Hayhow and Levy 1989). The authors refer to first- and second-order change as described by Watzlawick et al. (1974) where first-order change focuses on altering the person's behaviours and second-order change focuses on changing attitudes. So it seemed that James needed to make both first- and second-order changes. First-order change would include improving the quality of fricatives, the use of new fricatives in connected and spontaneous speech, generalisation of this to life situations and maybe extending the range and competence of conversational strategies and skills.

James had already made some of these first-order changes by acquiring a new set of articulatory skills. It was necessary that he generalise them into the full range of social situations. A behavioural-cognitive model would seem appropriate and his EPG work to date fitted into this.

In our first meeting I was aware of a dilemma about whether to commence a behavioural programme, possibly paying more attention to the cognitive elements and if so how long we were likely to benefit from that approach, because it quickly became apparent that James also had a series of second-order goals that would need to be addressed. He saw his lack of friends, girlfriend, intimacy and camaraderie as being brought about by his communicative style, which was passive, retiring, shy and reclusive.

It seemed clear that this behaviour was in part the result of low self-esteem and his fear of rejection. When discussing assignments he repeatedly made comments such as 'Nobody would be interested in what I have to say, even if I said it well, because I'm not very interesting.' It was obvious that significant second-order change would be necessary to redress James' general unhappiness, specifically: increasing self-esteem, increasing his ability to initiate relationships, reducing the need to defend himself against relationships, the development of a less judgmental inner critic, less reliance on other people's judgements, increased confidence and consequent, on this, more openness, self-disclosure and enjoyment of conversations and relationships. Such changes would allow him to implement his new phonological behaviour and to benefit from it. Chicken and egg, so where to start? Here was someone who hadn't asked for general counselling and who had never worked in this way before. I was inclined to use behavioural and cognitive methods to bring about the first-order change followed by generic counselling to bring about second-order change. As the two models are so different I decided to spend the first eight weeks on a behaviour therapy programme paying attention to associated cognitive elements and that this would also allow me to get to know James and make some judgements about how he might work in a counselling framework. In view of his concreteness I also thought he might find it an acceptable way into a less directed style of working. So the behavioural therapy would stabilise and generalise the existing new articulatory behaviour while the cognitive elements would focus on removing resistances to the new behaviour. At eight weeks we would review and maybe commence counselling in order to promote second-order change.

Formal assessments

In the early days of therapy I asked James to complete the Situation Avoidance Questionnaire (Johnson et al. 1963), the Rosenberg Test of Self-Esteem (Rosenberg 1965) and both self and ideal self characterisations. These were repeated towards the end of therapy and are discussed further later in the chapter but it is appropriate to look at the characterisations here.

Self-characterisation

> James is 29 years of age and single. He lives alone in his own house. James is a shy and reserved person who finds it difficult to instigate a conversation with strangers. His is, by profession, a librarian. He finds it difficult to converse with members of the opposite sex, which is why he has never had a long-term relationship with a girlfriend.

This is notably brief. We can see shyness, reluctance to initiate interactions, lack of relationships with women, his single status and the importance of his professional life to his identity. The first and last lines echo each other so we can bear in mind that this issue may have particular significance. I was particularly struck by his throwaway comment as he handed over the characterisation: 'It's short because there's not much to me.' The following week I asked him to do an ideal characterisation:

James is a hard working, friendly person who is easily approachable and dependable. He is a smart and friendly person who is easy to talk to. He is able to talk to anyone at the drop of a hat about anything and everything. He is very happily married with two very nice well behaved children. His interests include photography, philately, amateur dramatics and Karaoke singing. He is someone I feel you could approach with your problems and he would do his best to help. He is a valuable friend, respected colleague and wonderful dinner host.

The main themes here are an impressive ability to converse, longing for marriage and family, as well as wanting to be approachable, friendly and interesting to other people. There is a huge distance between current and ideal selves. The ideal self is super-skilled and able in all types of communication. It is slightly longer and more detailed than the self-characterisation. Certainly Karaoke didn't seem to fit at all with what I knew of him so far and hinted at a more extrovert part of his personality.

Major themes that emerged over the first three months

Self-esteem

This was low and there was some self-directed hostility. He described a critical and emotionally demanding mother. From an early stage in our work together I experienced James as having personal warmth and in no way experienced him as being shallow or having nothing to say. On the contrary, although it was hard to get him talking, his comments were useful and honest and interesting. When I confronted him with this in session 7, he looked embarrassed and said I was probably just trying to encourage him.

Harsh inner critic

Our internalised self-dialogue is influenced in our early life by those with whom we interact, primarily parents and other significant figures. Sometimes the voices are harsh and critical and slow to praise. Webster and Poulos (1989) call this 'negative self-talk'. It was not clear where this harsh inner critic came from: possibly from an overcritical mother or it may have been goal-induced. James had very high expectations of himself and continually measured himself as failing against his ideals.

Loneliness

James quickly admitted to being lonely. He had moved into his own house in order to force himself to develop a circle of friends but this hadn't happened. He had some friends at work although nobody with whom he really felt close or in whom he felt able to confide. Since starting therapy he had begun going to the local pub, although he spoke of it as an effort of will rather than as a pleasure. He expressed a longing for a girlfriend but always in terms of finding a girlfriend, getting married and then having children. The possibility of different types of relationships, or several relationships first, was not considered.

Goals/rewards

As part of the behaviour therapy I wanted to ascertain his attitude to praise in order to find out what sort of positive reinforcement would be acceptable. He had a strong tendency to negate praise with such thoughts as: 'People who say nice things about me are wrong or not good judges of character' and 'If Sara (the EPG therapist) gives me praise I pretend to accept it but I really think she's just trying to be nice to me.' James appeared to be extremely goal oriented and to have his life strictly mapped out against a timetable or series of goals that included promotion, getting married, having children and travelling. He expressed strong feelings of falling behind on this and consequently lived with a constant sense of time running out. By continually measuring his progress along this timetabled route against that of members of the public with whom he came into contact, he saw himself as failing. Thus he lived with the consequent disappointment, sadness and dread of a future that he saw as merely holding more of the same disappointment.

Grief

There was much unexpressed grief for his father who died 13 years earlier. He had never spoken to anyone about his father's death. He also appeared to be grieving for what he saw as the repressed areas of his own personality, such as intimate, spontaneous and carefree feelings and actions, as well as for what he saw as his own wasted life so far.

Control

He was much more comfortable when things were tightly structured in communicative situations and felt uncomfortable with general conversations and spontaneous speech. Parties were a nightmare. He was most at ease when giving set pieces of information as he might at work. He was very organised and neat in appearance. Initially he needed specific questions and feedback from me to initiate dialogue but he became much happier with the open-ended structure of sessions – at least, he never overtly challenged this way of working. James said he would like to be more spontaneous but he always left others to take the initiative in relationships and conversations, hoping for the other person to speak first. This was certainly reflected in our sessions. The notion that his own behaviour might affect other people's behaviour towards him was a new and important one for him.

Depression

He didn't use this word for a long time, but spoke of a 'downward spiral'. He became depressed two or three times a week but could lift himself out of minor depressions by doing something he liked. Major ones just got worse. Depressions were triggered by holidays and long periods of time spent alone. He admitted eventually to suicidal thoughts. 'If I thought things couldn't get any better than this, or if I lost my job, I wouldn't want to carry on.'

Assertiveness

He showed a tendency towards passive aggression and had very few strategies for dealing with taunting, mimicry and so forth. He had fantasised about confronting aggressors but never did; instead he withdrew and felt angry inside but didn't express it. This was a pattern from schooldays. His fantasy of the aim of confrontation was to make perpetrators feel small like he did. He didn't see a need for other strategies. He was desperate to minimise his lisp in front of these aggressors and said he wished his friends had stood up for him in school.

Therapy, progress and change

The behavioural programme

We had completed the behavioural programme. During preliminary hierarchy construction, the factors affecting anxiety levels emerged as:

- the extent to which the conversation was structured: he was happier in a highly structured dialogue such as those he encountered at work – he referred to these as his 'patter'. He was very anxious during free ranging conversations and avoided them, and had a mental checklist of topics he could bring up in the form of questions that he would systematically work through when he was attempting to make conversation;

- how well he knew the listener: strangers were easier, people in authority were hard;
- sex of listener: women were easier because they were more patient. Talking to women his own age or whom he found attractive was anxiety provoking;
- attitude of listener: the qualities of kindness, patience and encouraging body language all helped.
- relationship to listener: work situations were easier because the majority of his confidence came from his professional status. Any self-esteem he did have seemed linked to work, although he frequently verbalised regret at this state of affairs.

We had completed small assignments in the work environment, James spontaneously moving himself up a stage when he'd successfully completed a task. We had to clarify what would count as success. James' criteria were initially impossibly high but we settled on 80% of fricatives being accurate for a given period. He quickly grasped the elements of this approach and took responsibility for his own learning. We clarified his goals and expectations and identified top and bottom of a speaking situation hierarchy. Motivation was very high. I taught him the principles of desensitisation and he quickly grasped the application of this, inventing assignments, moving himself up and down a hierarchy and adjusting variables as required.

The cognitive issues

I was becoming increasingly aware of thought patterns that seemed to make life difficult for James. He showed rigidity of thinking, with a marked tendency to see things as black or white. Examples of such thoughts were: 'other people judge me negatively; everything would be OK if my speech was OK; life is a one track path; there is a time clock ticking away; I won't travel or try to fulfil any of my dreams until I have a special girlfriend, because I want those moments to be perfect; groups of people will leave me out; other people don't like me.' At the same time, he was beginning to see that his own behaviour might be affecting how people reacted to him. When debriefing on assignments, James frequently referred to himself as being shallow, not worth talking to, having nothing to say and having no opinion that was worth other people listening to. These thoughts prevented him from experimenting with his new speech because he did not feel that anyone would want to listen to him, regardless of whether his speech was good or bad.

My original thoughts were confirmed as it became more and more apparent that any behavioural programme would fall short of helping James significantly. Perfect speech would not make him any less lonely; we needed a different approach. In our early sessions James was unforthcoming and passive and needed a great deal of prodding to voice his thoughts, feelings and ideas. This gradually changed and he became much more responsive. So at eight weeks we mutually agreed to change tack and embark on counselling with the understanding that we were unlikely to focus on his speech in the way we had until now.

Counselling

At three months

By now there was a marked change in demeanour in sessions. James was more relaxed: he expressed a longing for change and to express hidden elements of his personality. He was honest in sessions and began volunteering information and ideas and to self-disclose. He was very co-operative when it came to carrying out experiments, becoming less passive generally. He spontaneously used metaphor, one in particular seemed powerful for him – a picture of the sun being kept behind a wall and the wall's imprisonment of that sun. At various stages we used empty chair techniques and written dialogues to promote a conversation between the wall and the sun and thus look at and resolve some of the conflict between them.

At four months

James hit a low point, triggered by a holiday. Holidays were times to be feared because they meant increased time alone at home and induced feelings of loneliness and hopelessness. They inevitably led to depression. At such times the 'timetable' loomed large. He told me he had had suicidal thoughts in the past though now kept these at bay by the prospect of change, '. . . but if I thought nothing would change then I wouldn't want to go on with it.' I had already obtained permission from James to contact his GP if we ever thought it advisable and at this low point I gave him my home phone number with the invitation to phone me if things felt too hard to bear. He did say that as his speech was improving and he was hopeful for the future, he didn't feel the need to take up either. He spoke of a desire to travel but said he was prevented from doing this by having no one to go with as he couldn't even contemplate joining a group of strangers for the fear of not being accepted and being lonely in a strange place. He was also waiting until he had a special partner to share it with so the experience would be perfect. Consequently he had never been abroad though he very much wanted to (it was one of his goals) and financially it was well within his reach.

At five months

At this time formal articulation therapy with Sara ended and James was seeing her on review. He was using the new /s/ outside clinic and reported success 60% of the time, with 35% of the time some dentalised fricatives. He thought that he reverted back to old later-alised sounds 5% of the time. He was finding listening to himself on tape easier and now found it a useful tool for checking accuracy. He reported slowing his rate of speech (he used to talk fast so the listener couldn't focus on the bad sounds) and said this helped accurate production of new sounds. Telephones were reported as being easier, because he no longer anticipated being quizzed about his intelligibil-ity. He was generally less worried about intelligibility in social situa-tions. He handled the end of articulation therapy well and round about this time attributed a reduced frequency of depression to his increasing ability to maintain his own opinions. He said other people's points of view would previously have overwhelmed his own. He used the metaphor of a wheelbarrow getting overladen with the conflicting views and opinions of others until it toppled over, sending him into a depression. In addition he could now, at least in fantasy, contemplate joining social groups although he was reluctant to do so in reality. However, real life relationships were stronger, less fragile than before and he had gained more casual friends and acquain-tances. He had more self-respect and felt he was receiving more respect from others, and that he was more approachable and more likely to volunteer his opinions rather than waiting to be asked all the time. He was generally getting more satisfaction out of conversa-tions. He had taken part in Karaoke sessions at the pub and said he had a better outlook on life, 'I laugh more, am more laid back.' The ticking clock was still there but people at work had told him he was 'coming out of himself'. During sessions he was more positive and optimistic and wanted to talk about asking a girl out. There was much more use of humour: he had a very engaging sense of humour and, though he only used it occasionally, I enjoyed it when he did. James was less passive and continuing to employ more self-disclosure in sessions. He also looked more relaxed.

At 1 year

There had been highs and lows in James' therapy. He felt he was still losing ground in the Great Life Plan and this bothered him greatly. From the transcripts below we can obtain a flavour of the issues that were important at this time. He displayed much bitterness towards his younger self for what he saw as taking the wrong path and making the decision to withdraw and shun friendships. For this reason he very much blamed his younger self for his present, expecting that younger self to have acted with confidence and wisdom. He was quite unrelenting in his condemnation of this unwise, unconfident child.

D I can understand you're saying there are some things you are hoping I don't ask about. What is it about these things that's worrying?

J Because I think some questions necessitate me to re-evaluate my past, which I'm not wholly happy about. It's a similar principle to the time clock, it's a form of evaluation.

D Mm.

J And I'm not happy with where I am at the moment.

J Or indeed what choices I've made in the past.

D Mm. Isn't that sort of implying the re-evaluation is going to make you feel worse about things?

J It does! (laughs)

D Have you thought about the possibility that re-evaluation might make you feel happier about it?

J Er, well I can only refer to my own experiences and, generally speaking, re-evaluation is a sad time rather than a joyous occasion since I tend to focus on the negative issues rather than the positive ones.

D OK, I think what's happening here with us is that we're using the word 're-evaluate' in different ways. You're using it in the sense of thinking about and judging the past while I'm meaning, yes, look at the past, but look at it in a different way from the way you're used to doing. Are you with me . . . that's a bit tortuous?

J Right.

D So in some ways I'm trying to challenge the way you evaluate your past at the moment.

J Well from our discussions I think that would be my initial intention although I always seem to go back to the same answers.

D Which are . . .?

J Non-complimentary. Negative.

D Are those negative evaluations about things that have happened to you or about things you've done to yourself? Do you distinguish between those two?

J No.

D You lump them into one category.

J Yes.

D Maybe that's one of the ways in which you make things difficult for yourself and in which you're quite hard on yourself. I'm all for us taking responsibility about what happens to us in our lives but some things we can't be responsible for . . . things that other people did, or if you get ill, that's not your fault, things that happened when you were a young child aren't your fault.

J But aren't they closely related, how you react to your circumstance?

D Yes, of course. I can't help thinking that a lot of the things you've told me about yourself happened when you were really young, like being teased by other kids at school.

J But even at that time the choices open to me were different weren't they? I didn't have to take the path I did. If I made a conscious or subconscious effort to act in a certain way then I could also have made a conscious effort to act in a different way.

D In theory, I don't know that stands up to everything. I mean if you've got . . . um . . . well, let's say you were watching a young child the same age as you . . . 8? . . . 9?

J Yeah, 8 or 9.

D Well if you were watching an eight year old being teased in a play-ground and you saw that eight year old go off, be very quiet by himself somewhere and feel very hurt . . . well we could say he could have done something different but we're not surprised that he didn't. We can understand that child pulling away from people and going to hide for a bit . . .?

J Well . . . like flicking a coin. There were two possible choices and I am of the opinion that I took the wrong one.

D Do you remember making a decision? Conscious or unconscious?

J I remember a sort of debate about it but not if it was at the time or subsequently. If I was to go back in time and see myself back in the playground I would be willing myself to take a different option.

D OK. And would you feel any sympathy towards that little boy for not being able to take a different option?

J Not as much as if I were watching someone else.

D Mmm? So you can't be as sympathetic to yourself as you would be to someone else?

J Yes.

D That doesn't seem very fair?

J [Long pause.]

D What's happening?

J I was just thinking perhaps it was because I was being lazy in not trying to improve the situation rather than sitting back and letting the world go by without me.

D Mm. Lazy . . .?

J Not prepared to put an effort in. And taking things too personally.

D Don't all children do that?

J Perhaps so, but I've tended to carry it on to my adulthood as well, which is something I'm not wholly proud of, although I don't see it's something I should apologise for.

D I agree . . . you were sounding pretty harsh and unforgiving and impatient with yourself just then. [Long pause.] Who might expect you to apologise?

J The part of me that's lonely.

D Right.

J . . . the part of me that's unhappy and the part of me that's trying to get out but can't.

D Mmm. So the part that's suffered as a result of what's happened.

J Yes.

D Mm . . . I'm not sure I agree that the little boy should have made a different decision, 'cause that's expecting a lot of a nine year old, but let's go along with it just for the minute . . . would you be able to feel any forgiveness towards him for making the wrong decision?

J [long pause] . . . well it's a *fait accompli* really and no good dwelling on 'I should have done this' all the time. However I er . . . I still wish that events had taken another course. [Long pause.]

D But they didn't.

J [Long pause.] No.

D And this is where you are right now . . .

At this point James was very quiet and close to tears. It felt like a deep acknowledgement of his present self and his earlier hostility had vanished. When I listened to the tapes in order to make the transcriptions I was even more aware of the long silences – nothing unusual in counselling, of course, but it struck me forcibly that, even after nearly a year of working together, I continually had to guard against our dialogue becoming an open question/answer format. James' passive role in conversations and relationships really pressured me to take a leading role, no matter how much I resisted. He still showed a marked tendency to think things through very carefully before verbalising a coherent, finished thought and was reluctant to think aloud. I was also becoming increasingly aware of how, at the beginning of sessions, even after a long period of working together, he never spoke first. I usually opened sessions by asking him if there was anything in particular he wished to talk about that day. He would nearly always decline and obviously thought this a strange manoeuvre. Around this time we reviewed how far we had come and I asked James to think about where he wanted to go from here. He deferred immediately to my superior wisdom and insight and said he would do whatever I thought was best. When I told him I did not have a master plan for his personality development stored somewhere in my head he was dreadfully surprised and when we talked it through he said he would need time to think about it. He still seemed excessively goal-oriented with much talk of ladders, scales, improvement and progression. This may have been a consequence of moving from a behavioural programme but I also believed it reflected James' own inherent need for structure.

At 15 months

In the summer of 1996 I made a personal decision to leave my post at the university and was aware this might affect James. It was important to handle this phase of our relationship well as he had recently taken the risk of letting me know that he 'couldn't imagine how he would manage without the sessions'. James was visibly shocked by the news that I would be leaving in six months' time. We talked through possible options and he told me he had always seen us tailing the sessions off gradually when I thought he needed to. This led us to revisit the territory of whether I carried some grand scheme for his happiness in my head. I was wary of interfering with the therapy process but it seemed a reasonable time to ask James to write something for this chapter, partly as a way of reviewing where we were and partly as a way of deciding how best we might use the remaining months. I asked him to write about what he felt had changed for him since we started. He wrote predominantly about his own response to counselling:

> When I was invited to go and speak with Diana I was just under the impression that Diana was someone who might be able to help me with my speech impediment. I had no idea in what form the meeting would take, but I had imagined that I would be hypnotised, and all my conscious and sub-conscious thoughts and phobias would be revealed, analysed and treated to create a 'new person'. I envisaged this re-birth would take a mere one or two sessions. I realised during our first meeting that this was not to be the format and the road to self-analysis, development and improvement was going to be a much harder route.

> When I met Diana my life revolved around work. My happiness and self-esteem revolved around my work and thus I became a workaholic. I thrived on hard work sometimes having two, three and sometimes four jobs at one time. However in my personal life I felt I had few close friends and I was prone to times of loneliness and despair and if work was not going well then I would fall into depression.

> There have been times in my life when I have seriously considered suicide but I was consoled by the idea that things could not get much worse and before I committed suicide I should reap the rewards of the money I had saved.

> I realised that in order to fully benefit from my meetings with Diana
> that I would have to be totally open and honest. This was far easier
> said than done since I had spent years ignoring, burying and
> concealing my problems.

By October 1996 James was taking the risk of talking much more easily and openly about his relationship with me and what the sessions meant to him. This seemed so different from the guarded person he had been when we met:

J . . . I was afraid of being ridiculed or leaving myself vulnerable to being ridiculed so that was the safe option, to keep quiet.

D Is it still the safer option?

J Umm . . . well the problem being that you are only the real, that you are only the, only the person that I would at this stage feel . . . er . . . secure about talking about them.

D Mm.

J I mean obviously, my mother's not changed, she's still the same and there's no one else I would feel close to in that, to be able to talk about everything.

D Mm. So at the moment I'm a safe person and there isn't anyone else who's available to you who's that safe.

J That's right. I mean because my mother's the only immediate family, primarily it would be a member of the family that you'd perhaps turn to, you'd have grown up with them and they'd shared similar experiences.

D Sometimes family members know where to hit.

J Yeah.

D For some people.

J . . . but if families are solid, say blood is thicker than water and if they are supportive and you can approach them, they'd be someone you could go to and feel safe and you wouldn't be ridiculed by them . . . but because I don't have any contact with my sisters then that road's closed.

D Mm. Do you ever see that friends might fulfil that need for you?

J Well . . . I can see that, yes, friendships could, but I've not made strong enough friendships for that. I mean when I was at school, there were strong friendships but your worries were different then and what you could talk about was different . . . but I've not . . . those friendships have not carried on into adult life . . . so I don't feel at ease being able to speak on certain matters with friends, not that close I'd consider going to them and airing my views.

D Can you imagine ever having a friendship that was that close?

J In the future or the present?

D The future. As a possibility . . .

J Er . . . It is something that I strive for, yes.

A few months earlier James had said he couldn't ever imagine being able to confide in a friend. I also asked him to try to identify what, for him, had been key moments in our work:

> There have been a number of key moments during the sessions. The most notable is the time I discussed my father. This had been the first opportunity I had had to talk about my feelings and regrets and in doing so to come to terms with the tragic loss of my father's death.
>
> I had been troubled for some time with the feeling that time was passing me by and I was not achieving my social ambitions. I have learnt to come to terms with the years I have been in a social void and the dismay I felt for the time passing me by has been alleviated. Prior to my meetings with Diana I had been subject to bouts of varying degrees of depression ranging from mild to deep. At these times I would tend to withdraw within myself and see everything in a negative perspective. Diana helped me to recognise the barrier which inhibited my happiness and which restrained me from allowing my old character to be re-born and combat the negative emotions.
>
> Diana has helped me to see life in a new and brighter perspective and by having a more open and friendlier personality uninhibited by the fear of torment and ridicule.

Although this is not a characterisation as such, if we compared the general style with that of the characterisation written a year earlier we can see how much more open and realistic it is and how much more self-awareness and disclosure there is. A more honest acknowledgement of the degree of unhappiness also comes through in the use of words like 'torment'. The way he referred to me made me feel he was still reluctant to completely relinquish the role of expert he had given me.

At 18 months

At this time James had a lot of trouble at work and was blocked in his bids for promotion. He applied for posts elsewhere and got an interview but not the job. Despite this, he did not end up being depressed, which he acknowledged as positive. He felt less dependent on work for his self-esteem and validation now that his social life had improved. He frequently talked of the new friends he had made at the pub and at a badminton class. He spoke of invitations to parties and took the big step of inviting some of these people round for a meal on his birthday. This took a lot of preparation within our sessions, for he was convinced no one would want to come. He was surprised when his invitation was so popular he had to run two sittings on different days! He was making conscious efforts to take the initiative in conversations and to reveal a little more of himself to people. He reported this as paying dividends almost immediately. It intrigued me that he always spoke of friends in the abstract and when I asked him about this he said it was less worrying to do so, because naming them and labelling them as friends seemed risky and presumptuous, in case they didn't want to think of themselves as his friends. I invited him to tell me about his friends, naming them and describing them, after which James said it actually felt quite nice to talk about them in that way.

Ending

It felt important to have a good ending because I didn't want James to feel abandoned and wanted to make sure he was ready and able to end. By this time we had done a lot of stocktaking along the lines of 'where have we come from?' 'where are we now?' and 'what do we want to achieve in the remaining time?' This appeared to be paying off until a student approached him with a request to interview him about the psychological effects of articulation disorders for her dissertation. Uncharacteristically he did not reply to two letters from her but did raise it in a session. He said he was pulled between wanting to offer something back, in recognition of the help he had had, while not really wanting to talk the issues through with a stranger. On further exploration, he felt that by reviewing things with her he would have to confront his past life and things he had already 'dealt with' and that this would make him sad. He was frightened about getting depressed again. I suggested that if this was the case then maybe those things were still issues and not 'dealt with' at all. I very much had the feeling that he needed to grieve for, and then let go of, what he saw as the wasted years. This led us to identify things he wished to take forward from his 'old life' into the future and things he wanted to leave behind. At first he was sceptical about finding anything worth salvaging but eventually he managed to identify a substantial list of things he deemed worth saving, in the form of personal qualities and hopes. We symbolically packed all these in a suitcase, to prepare him for his onward journey. The last few sessions were spent looking at how he saw the first months after the end of therapy and how he saw his life developing generally, all of which seemed realistic and even optimistic. James said the main feelings were anxiety at how he would manage without the sessions, also excitement at the thought of being his new self and seeing how life would go. He seemed much more tolerant of himself than he had been. In the last session he told me he'd booked a holiday in Canada with a woman friend, first time in an aeroplane, first time abroad. I asked him if he had any better understanding, looking back, of why I had not had his therapy, or a life plan mapped out for him. I knew this had been a difficult part of our work together and wondered whether he could make better sense of it now. He agreed that at the time he had been confused and angry at this, but now he felt it was a better way to work because the changes were more fundamental and he had some confidence about being able to deal with difficulties for himself when they came up. 'If you'd told me what sort of person to be, I don't think it would have lasted very long, and the first little knock I'd have wanted to come running back.' James promised to send me a postcard from Niagara Falls.

Evaluation

When I began to work with James I was unclear about which assessments would, in the end, prove to be most useful and therefore asked him to complete three short tests in between our early sessions; an avoidance/reaction questionnaire, self and ideal-self characterisations and the Rosenberg self-esteem scale. I was interested to know which of these, at the end of therapy, would feel to have most accurately reflected what had changed.

The self characterisation and ideal-self characterisation

I borrowed the ideas of self characterisation and ideal-self characterisation from personal construct theory because a characterisation gives access to important information at an early stage and by comparing the two, clear indications as to major areas of unhappiness/dissatisfaction. It pushes clients into thinking deeply in a way they may not have done before and is a useful concrete way into more open styles of working. On the downside, it asks a client to focus at a point in therapy when an exploratory, opening out mode may be more appropriate. Nevertheless it alerted me to some issues, and reinforced those impressions gleaned during early sessions. With the benefit of hindsight it seems that the two characterisations completed at the beginning of therapy did indeed offer reliable clues but I can now see that, in one sense, this information can be superficial. This depends on the person doing the characterisation of course. My intention was to obtain two more characterisations at the end of therapy because comparing before and after characterisations may give a clear sense of how things had changed for him, not only from the content of the piece but also from the style of it, language, length etc. I did ask James to do this but he never produced one, possibly because he was also writing other, similar pieces at this stage, more directly concerned with the process of his therapy and I did not want to confuse him nor be too demanding about having almost identical information put into exactly the style I wanted.

The Rosenberg self-esteem scale

At the beginning I was not familiar with self-esteem measures and was influenced by ease of administration, availability and ease of completion for the client. The Rosenberg scale asks the client to rate himself on a scale of 1–4 in five negative and five positive statements pertaining to self-esteem. There are no scoring sheets or standardisation charts, so the test is a way of recording information rather than interpreting that information. The use of such tests relies on the counsellor spotting trends and movements on repeated testings. I understand that this is an accepted format for tests in social science disciplines although for us it is a less familiar way of approaching assessment. James' before and after ratings are given below in Table 6.1, where B = before therapy, A = after.

If we compare before and after ratings, there are changes in a positive direction in nine out of the 10 items, with one item remaining static. The most marked changes were in items 4, 8 and 10 which moved by 2 degrees, indicating marked changes in self-respect, a feeling of being able to do things as well as other people and a lessening in the feeling of being 'no good at all'.

Table 6.1: James' scoring of the Rosenberg Test of Self-Esteem

	strongly agree	agree	disagree	strongly disagree
1. I feel that I am a person of worth, at least on an equal plane with others	B	A		
2. I feel that I have number of good qualities	B	A		
3. All in all I am inclined to feel that I am a failure			B	A
4. I am able to do things as well as most people	A		B	
5. I feel I do not have much to be proud of		AB		
6. I take a positive attitude towards myself		A	B	
7. On the whole, I am satisfied with myself		A	B	
8. I wish I could have more respect for myself		B		A
9. I certainly feel useless at times			B	A
10. At times I think I am no good at all		B		A

A= at the start of therapy
B= towards the end of therapy.

Avoidance/reaction questionnaire

The use of this questionnaire reflects the behavioural nature of the early part of therapy. I have not reproduced the test sheet itself because speech and language therapists are familiar with it. In this test, the higher the avoidance score, the more the client avoids situations and the higher the reaction score, the more aversion there is to speaking situations in general. The overall scores were:

Before	After
Avoidance: 51	Avoidance: 36
Reaction: 76	Reaction: 69

If we look at the avoidance scores, there is a marked decrease with fewer situations being avoided and a decrease in the degree of avoidance shown in a particular situation. In fact, by the end of therapy there were no responses that any longer indicated definite avoidance of speaking situations, although ambiguity was registered for a couple of situations. The decrease in reaction scores, although less dramatic than the avoidance scores, indicates both an increased level of enjoyment in some of the speaking situations and a decrease in the level of dislike towards others.

Direct feedback

In addition to the formal assessments, I want to mention the informal feedback I was picking up from James. In the latter part of therapy we did much talking through issues about what sort of things had changed for him and what he thought had brought those changes about. Sometimes I asked him to write these down and he always brought them in to show me. I was also alert to his gradually changing demeanour during the sessions themselves, his increasing use of humour, openness, as well as an increasingly realistic attitude, cheerful mood and generally optimistic attitude to the future.

To summarise, as a measure of change, the avoidance/reaction questionnaire was useful as a confirmation of a clinical impression, but the self characterisations, verbal feedback and observable changes in James' demeanour during the session felt like the methods that gave the broadest data and came closest to truly reflecting the essence of what was happening between us, changes that had taken place both in the dynamics of the session and in James' life outside the session as well as the meaning of those changes for him.

Writing up

I found this chapter very labour intensive to write as I kept pulling on a number of different models. I must have edited out as much text again as is presented here in an endeavour to thoroughly apply my theoretical knowledge. This is one danger of an eclectic approach, it's tempting to jump between models solely to make things fit. On the other hand one cannot unlearn what one knows and so I wrestled with concepts mainly from cognitive behaviour therapy (CBT), personal construct therapy (PCT), client-centred therapy and occasionally Gestalt, all of which contributed to my understanding of James and his problems.

The other difficulty in writing up a report of this nature is finding a way to organise the material in such a way as to summarise a complex relationship that has operated over 18 months and the subtle changes that have occurred in that time. To allocate any client that amount of time would be a luxury in today's National Health Service. Even in a university environment I was not free of constraints: in order to justify seeing clients at all, I either had to get teaching time out of them, or a research paper. Even so, the demands of satisfying research quotas these days don't fit well with long-term therapy and I was certainly aware of a pressure, both from myself and others, to get on with both the therapy and writing the case history, so I could start something new. I had to repeatedly check any tendency for this to interfere with James' actual therapy.

Articulation therapy with adults: transfer and maintenance

There was almost nothing in the literature about the transfer of articulation skills in a remedial programme with adults to help me plan James' therapy. With children it seems it is rarely necessary to work on transfer in such a structured way, it being commonly accepted that children are likely to generalise spontaneously into outside situations, 'Once the child has attained adequate control of the defective phonetic sounds and phoneme sequences he will incorporate them into his own speech, with the minimum of guidance, and in all normal linguistic sequences' (Morley 1969, also Elbert et al. 1990). In fact Elbert et al. then go on to say that when children do not spontaneously generalise, only a small number of treatment examples are necessary to achieve it.

The literature on generalisation in adults refers primarily to fluency, where it is commonly regarded as a response in its own right in a behavioural training programme (Ingham 1980) and to a much lesser extent in aphasia, although the latter texts are mainly concerned with generalisation across linguistic categories and not with generalisation into other contexts. In any case it would be foolish to apply the processes of a brain-damaged population to a non-brain-damaged one. Whereas some adults may be able to make some progress in generalisation on their own, most need help and so transfer and the maintenance of new skills are familiar issues for therapists who work with adults.

Compared with what followed, behaviour therapy did not figure largely in my overall management of James but the dilemma of where to start, as well as the potential problem of long-term skill decay, did give me much cause to pause and consider in the early stages, so I will revisit some of my thinking at that time. The question of how best to help people transfer skills between environments invokes a debate that has continued for nearly 100 years in educational circles (Wellington 1993). Transfer is defined by Glaser (1962) as the ability to utilise one's learning in situations that differ, to some extent, from those in which learning occurs; alternatively, transfer may refer to the influence of learning in one situation or context upon learning in another situation or context (Ausubel 1969). Lave (1988) felt that 'when we investigate learning transfer across situations, the results are consistently negative'. Even if skills do transfer within an educational context, it cannot be assumed they will transfer from the educational context to the world outside. It is no good having a large number of general concepts or skills if they are only partially understood. Such learning is quickly forgotten because it is not fully meshed in with other, securely anchored parts of our cognitive battery. Once again I found most help when I looked to literature on the transfer of fluency techniques. Transfer in a speech and language therapy setting is usually achieved by behavioural methods although Hayhow and Levy (1989) reject the static concept of maintenance of fluency in favour of what they feel is the more optimistic view of change and development inherent in personal construct theory. They find this more appealing than the behaviourist concept of maintenance, which implies keeping things the same. I agree with this yet at the same time it may be one respect in which articulatory transfer differs from fluency transfer because one would not expect an articulation, once well established, to be destabilised by external factors. We would expect the target behaviour to be maintained under varying conditions (Van Riper 1973) except in any transitional period before the behaviour has been stabilised, when one would expect to see variation as a result of stresses. However, Sharkey and Manning (1987) were unable to be conclusive about the effects of emotional arousal and increased speaking rate on children's newly learned /r/ productions.

In terms of the social and psychological consequences of the core speech disorder, the closest practical parallel for adults with chronic articulation disorders would also seem to be with fluency, although I acknowledge that we cannot say for certain which features the two disorders share and which are unique to each group. In a discussion on PCT and relapse, Hayhow and Levy (1989) point out that '. . . just as the stuttering/fluency construct remains one of the most highly elaborated ways of making sense of self in relation to others, it may govern that person's interpersonal behaviour'. I expected James's speech behaviour to have been just as crucial for him in developing a sense of self.

In fluency work it is common practice to follow a behavioural transfer programme that incorporates elements of cognitive therapy, in order to establish and maintain a fluency technique. It is also common practice to incorporate elements of PCT to change the client's attitudes and ways of relating to the world. A common way of organising intervention would be to initiate the behavioural programme, supplemented by cognitive work and then, as insight develops or if behavioural plus cognitive approaches are not as successful as hoped, to introduce PCT. Sometimes all three therapies are used simultaneously, with single sessions containing elements of all three, but I wanted to avoid this as it can be muddling for client and therapist. Instead we used the format already described, an eight-week broadly behavioural programme followed by longer-term counselling. So with James I used an orthodox fluency model but did not use PCT to provoke second-order change, choosing instead a generic counselling approach. However, self characterisations and ideal self characterisations were used as an assessment tool and a way of acquiring information at an early stage, and the concept of first- and second-order change was useful. I also kept the two models temporally separate, using a format of two discrete blocks of therapy.

Implications for children with 'minor' articulation disorders

Lisping negatively influences the judgement of adult audiences. When asked to rate adult male lispers on the five attributes of speaking – ability, intelligence, education, masculinity and friendship – judges rated the speakers more negatively than they did non-lispers (Mowrer et al. 1978). Silverman (1976) found that an adult with a lateral lisp will be evaluated by his peers as handicapped and urged that children with the condition should be treated as early as possible, a view with which I concur. Mowrer et al. (1978) also point out that although listener evaluations may change on extended social contact with the lisper, many vital decisions are made about people on first impressions: job interviews, introductions, brief social contacts and so forth, and hence lisping can seriously jeopardise employment and social opportunities. This ties in with James' experience. He had reacted to the negative evaluations of others, and to some extent had internalised them, by withdrawing as much as possible from social interaction and suffering the consequences of isolation. Certainly, if intervention had been available to him as a child, James could have been saved many unhappy years and maybe would not have needed 18 months of therapy as an adult.

Chapter 8
Two hypnotherapy studies

ALLISON PENNINGTON

Introduction – case history 1: treatment of articulation problems and dysphonia in Parkinson's disease – case history 2: control of spastic dysphonia in a 40-year-old male – hypnotic techniques used in the case reports.

Introduction

Breaking a leg is probably not the best way of ensuring that one moves to a new professional field, but that was the way it happened to me. After the skiing trip from hell had rendered me horizontal for seven months I was faced with two choices: to wallow in the depths of despair and look forward only to my next mealtime or to use the time profitably and pursue an area of medical science that had long held an interest for me: hypnotherapy and its potential applications within the field of speech and language therapy.

This field had always held an interest for me mainly, I think, due to my own personal awareness of the power of the mind. The old saying 'you can if you think you can' had always struck a chord with me and over the past 10 years, personal experience had taught me the importance of a focused and strong mind and of learning to empower oneself in the face of life's knocks and in this way find a new and refreshing freedom. To this end, as soon as the crutches would permit I hopped down to Birmingham and completed a three-day course under the auspices of Mr Samuel Abudarham, himself a speech and language therapist. My conclusions? An interesting course that set my mind in motion about the wide implications which hypnotherapy might have for our profession, but I felt it wasn't enough. The basics were there but I considered that further training was essential for a powerful and potentially dangerous therapy.

Enquiries with the Royal College of Speech and Language Therapists put me in touch with the Association for the Practice of Hypnotherapy in Speech and Language Therapy. On joining this association I received little in the way of correspondence and was once again disillusioned to learn that a three-day course was also all that was considered necessary in order for me to use hypnosis with any of my patients.

So I decided to look elsewhere and based on the 'where there's a will there's a way' philosophy, began to attend a few weekend seminars run by the Department of Psychiatry at the University of Sheffield, incognito to start with as there was a definite feeling at this time that these lectures, never mind courses, were the prerogative of doctors, dentists and psychologists.

However, in true Pennington tradition, I persevered delicately but firmly, believing strongly that just because it has always been done that way, it doesn't mean it has to carry on like that. By the end of the year I had been offered a place on the diploma course in clinical hypnosis.

The course ran for one year, covering eight weekends, 72 clinical hours, four case studies, two essays and numerous hours staring at a computer screen. Intensive but well worth it when I graduated with distinction. During the year I used hypnotherapy with a variety of patients, notably vocal disorders, stammerers, cerebral vascular disease and Parkinson's disease. I have also been working with hypnotherapy in the communication therapy department of the Royal Hallamshire Hospital.

So, where do I go from here? Well, I have recently been accepted on to the Masters component to the diploma course, which I began in September of this year, and will be undertaking a study as part of this, looking specifically at hypnosis and psychogenic voice disorders. The rest . . . well, who knows? Certainly there is a huge need for research into the applications within the field of speech and language therapy of this interesting and, to my mind, very effective therapy.

Case history 1: treatment of articulation problems and dysphonia in Parkinson's disease

Description of the problem

Mrs W, aged 74, was referred by her general practitioner for assessment and treatment of the articulatory dysarthria and dysphonia associated with Parkinson's disease, an illness caused by depigmentation and reduced dopamine content in the basal ganglia of the brain. The initial diagnosis was made in 1989. Presenting difficulties were poor intelligibility due to slow, slurred articulation, a harsh, strangled voice and jerky, sporadic breath control. The referral agent also reported that problems were intensified when Mrs W became anxious, an emotion she felt with increasing regularity as she watched her bodily and vocal musculature deteriorate and as she experienced a growing aversion to socialisation. She also indicated an intense frustration due to the recent necessity of intervention by the family over her physical and communication needs. She felt that others were beginning to talk for her, an activity that she had always valued and enjoyed.

Personal details

Mrs W had always been a bright, outgoing person who enjoyed every day to the full. She lived with her husband whom she described as 'a little mean at times', and had one daughter and two grandchildren, also living. Mrs W had one older sister, living locally, and a younger one abroad. Throughout her working life Mrs W nursed the elderly and in her spare time she was a keen countryside walker. Other hobbies included listening to classical music and painting. During the therapy period, daughter S underwent a vocal cord operation and Mrs W's elder sister was given a diagnosis of lung carcinoma – both anxiety-provoking situations for Mrs W.

Relevant investigations and formal assessment

Case history

This was taken on initial contact with Mrs W and included questions designed to gain both factual and emotional information from Mrs W's life. It also aimed to establish a motivation for therapy. A sample is shown below:

- When was your initial diagnosis?
- What situations and which people seem to make your voice

and articulation – worse/better?
- What's the one wish that you'd like to come true?

Formal speech and language therapy assessments

- A tape recording was taken of speech output in natural conversation prior to, and on completion of, each session of therapy. On each of these occasions, the same person, a non-linguist, was asked to give an auditory rating of overall speech intelligibility on a 1 to 5 scale. The person rating had never previously met Mrs W.

- A specialised auditory analysis of voice phonation, prosody, breath control and overall intelligibility was provided by a university centre for clinical communication disorders. Two recordings were submitted, one of conversational output prior to hypnotherapy and the other after hypnotherapy. The specialist was unaware of the correct sequence of the tapes.

- The Robertson Dysarthria Profile (Robertson 1982) was administered before and after therapy in order to pinpoint which areas within the general categories of intelligibility, voice quality and respiration were significantly contributing to any improvement or regression seen. The following components were assessed: maintenance of exhalation/inhalation; phonation; facial musculature; diadokochinesis, articulation and prosody. The profile included an analysis by the speech and language therapist of these components using the following rating scale:

1.   Poor
2.   Fair
3.   Good
4.   Normal

Mrs W scored poorly in tasks testing facial musculature, phonation, prosody and inhalation/exhalation.

Hypnotic susceptibility testing

From an initial session which indicated that Mrs W was going to enjoy and find relaxation easy, the 'Is it possible?' protocol (Margolin et al. 1992) was administered in order to establish the most effective channel for induction and therapy. This suggested that Mrs W found all modalities easy to experience, the only difficulty found was that of cloud flotation. It was therefore decided that a multi-modality approach would be used if appropriate.

Management

The case history revealed that Mrs W had been a worrier through-out her life, especially where her family was concerned. Considering the circumstances of her sisters, the low priority given to relaxation, the experience of loss of control over life and the suggestion that output deteriorated with increasing anxiety, the aims of therapy were originally to see

- whether output improved with deep relaxation and traditional communication therapy techniques within hypnotherapy, and
- to give back some form of confidence and control even if this could only be done through ego strengthening and autohypnosis, and not via an improvement in speech output. However it quickly became evident that Mrs W was a good hypnotic subject, capable of experiencing imagery along various channels and so, based on a strong personal belief that the mind is capable of re-stimulating external and internal bodily functions, it was jointly decided to add visualisation techniques to therapy (Simonton et al. 1978), to focus upon areas of damage, repair and subsequent health. Mrs W's existing knowledge of anatomy was also of significance in the choice of this technique.

Plan and description of therapy

A verbal contract of six sessions plus one review session was negotiated with Mrs W. Two aims of therapy were discussed – firstly to reduce anxiety, which seemed to be contributing to a harsh voice and slowed, dysarthric speech, and secondly, to give some control over phonatory and respiratory apparatus back to Mrs W. This would be achieved mainly by hypnotherapy techniques but these would on occasion be combined with traditional speech and language methods (Abudarham 1991). Mrs W was taught relaxation techniques through hetero- and autohypnosis and was further instructed in the visualisation of her malfunctioning and subsequently appropriately functioning speech musculature. Traditional breathing techniques were taught whilst in hypnosis aimed at strengthening the voice. Attempts were made to identify situations that created significant anxiety and these were mostly found to be associated with Mrs W's newly diagnosed sister.

Details of hypnotherapeutic intervention

Session 1

Mrs W was shown how to relax via her breathing, a concept that was completely new to her. She naturally closed her eyes and followed instructions to breathe in through the nose and out through her mouth, keeping the outward breath steady. Visualisation of a candle flame was used to ensure this breath control. At the end of this brief initial session, Mrs W reported that she felt 'wonderful and so relaxed'. At this point an explanation was given of the connection between relaxing the muscles and the ease and efficiency with which ensuing tasks are then done. The label of hypnosis was then introduced, defined and described in terms of its ability to further deepen relaxation and to bypass the critical mind. Potential fears regarding the forthcoming treatment were included (Waxman 1989) but Mrs W displayed only a keenness to commence therapy. Before leaving, Mrs W was asked to rehearse the breathing technique at home when convenient. A good rapport had been established and positive signs of a good trance subject seen.

Session 2

Mrs W arrived with the expectation of being hypnotised. She had been rehearsing the breathing technique over the week and felt 'somehow calmer'. Due to her natural propensity to eye closure, an eye fixation procedure was not used but induction proceeded with the attention being placed on the inhalation/exhalation of breath and on the word 'relax' paced with exhalation. Further suggestions were made of progressive relaxation, along with a request that Mrs W locate any bodily tension and ascribe a symbolic colour to it. A colour red was reported particularly around the chest and neck and so it was suggested that this could be released within each outward breath in the form of a coloured mist. When this had been completed Mrs W reported that the colour seen was now blue. Whilst deeply relaxed, suggestions were made that during the ensuing week, prior to speaking, Mrs W would keep her sentences short and ensure adequate air for their expression. Further suggestions aimed at ego strengthening and confidence building were added, with a reminder of how relaxation would help all of Mrs W's muscles work more efficiently, particularly those of her mouth, tongue, chest and neck. Mrs W was then reminded of the routine for self-hypnosis and this was rehearsed whilst still in trance. She was finally alerted using a 5 to 1 upwards count and then asked to demonstrate her self-hypnosis routine. Use was made of the valuable time just after alerting to further suggest the connection between relaxed muscles and ease of speech.

Session 3

Induction proceeded as described with the addition of a hand levitation (Erikson 1923) to deepen as trance seemed light. Coupling was also used to this end 'It is sinking down now . . . On to the chair. And as it does so . . . Are falling into a deeper, deeper sleep' (Waxman 1989). From here Mrs W was asked if there was anything troubling her as it was suspected that there might be. She immediately began to talk about her sister who had deteriorated during the week and of her daughter who was due to have an operation. Mrs W became distraught, markedly tense and again gave the colour red to symbolise this. At this point the planned session was abandoned and immediate ego strengthening suggestions were commenced, acknowledging her pain and focusing upon the importance of building up her own inner reserves and regaining some control over life in order to help herself to cope at this time. Mrs W was then relaxed again using the vapour technique and word 'focus'. Her colour then symbolically changed to green and thus she was reminded of the standard techniques of sentence shortening and breath control prior to alerting.

Session 4

Mrs W arrived in a happier frame of mind as her sister's condition had stabilised and her daughter's operation had been a success. She had been working on her hypnosis and speech therapy combination techniques and felt that her output was improved for up to five hours after each session. Her husband had also begun to remind her to practise them and commented on her improvement, which thrilled Mrs W.

The usual induction routine was used and Mrs W went deeply into trance. She used a previously taught ideomotor finger response to indicate when her trance was deep. At this point she was asked to remain in trance, but to open her eyes and have a good look at the picture being held up in front of her, which was a simplified line drawing of the oral, tongue, neck and chest musculature. From here use was made of indirect suggestion and metaphor (Erikson 1923) as a means of introducing the idea of visualisation of the phonatory and articulatory muscles. For example, 'You know I used to have a patient who also had Parkinson's disease and she found that her voice and speech improved when she started to visualise her speech muscles working smoothly and efficiently'. A further explanation was given of how thought can affect physical body parts (for example tensing of muscles, sexual arousal, blushing) and the suggestion added that the visualisation task would become easier with each attempt.

The visualisation

Using Mrs W's natural skills to the full, she was asked to paint a visual picture in her mind of her own damaged phonatory and articulatory musculature. Indirect suggestions were made of feeling, seeing and hearing the impulses coming from her brain as a result of her own positive thoughts of repair. It was further suggested that impulses took the form of white light energy running down her nerve channels, removing any tension blockages and entering her damaged musculature, bringing warmth, revitalisation and restimulation. In this way, the appropriate musculature would begin to work efficiently again without fault or hesitation. An ideomotor response was given when this had been achieved. Further ego strengthening suggestions were added regarding Mrs W's corresponding increase in confidence and control and instructions for using these techniques within autohypnosis were repeated.

Post-hypnotic suggestion

Prior to alerting, a trigger phrase was introduced in order to cut down on the lengthy induction procedure in future sessions. Mrs W was informed that, because she had become so skilled in hypnosis, all that was now necessary was the phrase 'You can go all the way' delivered by my voice alone. On alerting the trigger was rehearsed with success. The immediate post-alerting period was again used to further reinforce belief in the power of thought over bodily workings when one of Mrs W's arms began to shake and she was successfully able to stop it by repeating the instruction 'stop' in her mind and focusing on the arm. Again, Mrs W reported feeling 'smashing' as a result of the session.

Session 5

Mrs W arrived in a positive mood and again reported a significant improvement in her speech, also commented upon by her husband and some family friends. She had continued to do her autohypnosis over the week and believed this to be responsible for her progress. Her purse had been stolen midweek and, using her autohypnosis, she had been able to remain calm. She and her husband had also discussed the possibility of visiting her sister in the new year. The post-hypnotic trigger was given and Mrs W went swiftly into trance. She was again asked to 'paint' the oral, neck and chest musculature in her mind and to visualise the white light energy entering as previously described. On asking how the preparations made her feel, Mrs W replied 'Great, positive and confident, more my own self again.' These feelings were then anchored (Bandler and Grindler 1979) and she was again invited to use the visualisation/anchoring routine within autohypnosis at any appropriate time. The additional suggestion was made that, the more she did so, the more improvement there would be in speech output, confidence and control. Prior to alerting, the concept of an end to therapy was delicately introduced, informing her that next week would be the last session. It was made clear that Mrs W was ready for this because of progress made in speech output and her significant gain in confidence. As it was not deemed appropriate to completely sever relations at this stage, Mrs W was placed on review for a month. Prior to the alerting procedure it was suggested that Mrs W visualise a tree that had been planted in the early days of therapy and that was now beginning to bear fruit, a metaphor of her improved intelligibility. The number of fruits were counted by Mrs W. There were 10.

Session 6

Mrs W was in a state of upset as her sister had lapsed into unconsciousness in the week and so the first part of the session was spent listening. When asked if she wanted to continue with the session, she replied 'yes' because it seemed to be doing her so much good. She had been using the techniques for 15 minutes every day since the previous week and had received further positive comments about her speech. On the trigger word Mrs W went immediately into trance and the visualisation techniques previously discussed were again rehearsed with an ideomotor response shown when completed. Other suggestions of easy speech and fluency were made using the metaphor of a reel of silk, plus further suggestions of vocal cord relaxation and an increase in articulation rate.

Similar ego strengthening suggestions associated with improved speech output were made and again anchored. Mrs W was asked when she might use this technique and replied 'at my sister's funeral'. Prior to alerting a final suggestion was made regarding how the unconscious mind would be working on further improvement of voice quality and articulation in the days and weeks to come and finally the tree of improvement was again visualised. The number of fruits visualised had now risen to 19. Mrs W's speech output was then reassessed using the Robertson dysarthria profile.

Review session

Mrs W reported that her speech had remained much improved until two weeks previously when it had suddenly deteriorated again. She continued to give an account of her sister's death, which had occurred in the intervening period. She added that the GP had given her a new drug over the past two weeks. This was found to be Selegiline, a type B monoamineoxidase inhibitor (MAOI) designed to inhibit monoamineoxidase B in the synaptic cleft and so potentiate the effect of any dopamine released. Selegiline is also thought to inhibit the re-uptake of dopamine back into the neurones. The possibility of detrimental effects of Selegiline on oral musculature control is not well documented but is thought to be unlikely due to its mode of action. However, her intelligibility certainly seemed poorer and increasingly slurred and her voice was increasingly strained. Mrs W's trigger phrase was then given and the usual musculature visualisation techniques and ego strengthening suggestions were followed.

Summary

Mrs W was referred for treatment of the deterioration of articulatory dysarthria and dysphonia associated with Parkinson's disease. A detailed case history was administered along with traditional speech/language and hypnotherapy assessments. Six treatment sessions plus a review were undertaken utilising hypnotherapy as a means of experiencing deep relaxation, ego strengthening, visualisation and autohypnosis techniques. More traditional speech and language therapy techniques were also delivered while in trance, due to the belief that susceptibility to them and action upon them would be heightened under these circumstances. On reassessment after therapy, results showed a significant improvement in the areas assessed, with a corresponding improvement in confidence reflected in new events within the patient's life.

Case history 2: control of spastic dysarthria in a 40-year-old male

Description of the problem

Mr B was referred by the speech and language therapy department of a local general hospital for treatment of an undiagnosed voice disorder, described by the referring agents as a spastic dysphonia of indeterminate origin. This disorder has at its basis an abnormal adductor spasm of the vocal cords during phonation and may be associated with hyperfunctional voice, conversion reaction and neurological disorders. Presenting features were a consistently tremulous voice interspersed with frequent phonation breaks forming part of a tense and breathy laryngospasm, the major contributor to a bizarre strained and strangled voice quality. The referral agent had covered a number of traditional speech and language therapy techniques including syllable timed speech and breath control over a two-month period, without any improvement seen. They also reported that the problems were intensified when anxiety levels increased. Mr B felt his vocal difficulties to be the cause of his limited socialisation and forced dependence upon his parents, factors that caused him to feel intense frustration.

Personal details

Mr B was a very introverted man who was currently living back with his parents due to the need for support, particularly in communicative situations. He had never been married and found it very difficult to contend with social situations. At our initial meeting he reported that he only socialised with his parents and occasionally his younger brother, who was married with a family and lived locally. Mr B had spent most of his working life undertaking brief contracts for city companies. Hobbies included travelling and skiing in mountainous regions, all done alone. General pastimes tended to be avoided, particularly if they involved socialisation. Mr B lacked confidence in all areas of his life and felt extremely restricted. He presented as an uptight, anxious person, and interestingly perceived himself as anxious from time to time although not persistently in this state.

Formal assessment

Case history

This was taken on initial contact with Mr B and included questions designed to gain both factual and emotional information from his life. It also aimed to establish a motivation for therapy. Examples of the questions are:

- When was your initial consultation?
- What situations and which people seem to make your voice worse/better?
- What's the one wish you'd like to come true?

The history revealed a feeling of total inadequacy as a child. Mr B also revealed that very little affection was ever shown to him as a child and that such attention was constantly craved. In addition, he recalled frequently feeling neglected and believing that he was worthless as he watched his younger brother receive both attention and praise.

Medical investigations

Mr B was referred to the hospital ENT department for an indirect laryngoscopy examination. The consultant reported an anatomically normal larynx with fully mobile cords. The consultant and GP were also asked for any contraindications concerning the use of hypnotherapy, with none being raised.

Formal speech and language therapy assessments

The case sheet report form (Fawcus 1987, appendix 1) was used to record the therapist's vocal assessment findings before and after therapy on a 1–5 scale. Areas included pitch, breathiness, observed tension in voice, severity of dysphonia. A tape recording was made of vocal output in natural conversation and when reading a specific text prior to, and on completion of, each session of therapy. From here the episodes of laryngospasm per sentence were recorded. A phonetic transcription was also undertaken prior to, and on completion of, each therapy session to assess for a regular pattern of spasmodic sounds (Fawcus 1987, appendix 2). An external person, a non-linguist, was asked to give an auditory rating for the patient's vocal tremor at the start and on completion of overall therapy. This was given on a 1–5 scale. A biofeedback machine recorded pulse rate before and after each session in order to monitor developing relaxation skills.

Hypnotic susceptibility testing

From an initial session which indicated that Mr B was going to enjoy and find relaxation easy, the Creative Imagination Scale (Barber and

Wilson 1978) was administered in order to establish the most effective channel for induction and therapy. An overall score of 32 points out of a possible 40 was produced and, more importantly, it was discovered that Mr B found it relatively easy to imagine using visual, auditory and kinaesthetic channels. It was therefore decided that therapy would incorporate these modalities wherever it was appropriate to do so.

Plan of therapy

The case history revealed that Mr B had been an isolated individual since childhood and could not remember a time when he did not have the vocal problem. Initially, he could not recall any incident in his life when he had felt embarrassed or angry, which was a difficult statement to accept in view of the severity of the problem. As the interview progressed and rapport developed, however, he did admit that the vocal disorder sometimes caused these emotions to stir. In the light of these comments, the reported deterioration in vocal quality when stressed, the lack of awareness of a persistent anxiety state, the lack of self-confidence exhibited and indeed a suspected denial of the vocal severity, three aims of therapy were jointly discussed:

- to attempt to provide some form of alleviation for the laryngospasm via deep relaxation.
- to improve self-confidence and control even if only via ego strengthening techniques and autohypnosis, and not by an improvement in vocal quality.
- to address the suspected denial exhibited using exploratory and reconstruction methods, if appropriate, as a means of alleviating the symptoms. Such techniques were never actually needed in this case. Mr B was very happy for hypnotherapy to be used in order to work towards these goals. He had tried traditional techniques previously and had found them to be unhelpful.

It quickly became apparent that Mr B was a good hypnotic subject and could experience imagery along various channels, therefore it was jointly decided to utilise this capacity in the hypnotic techniques used.

Description of therapy

A verbal contract of six sessions at fortnightly intervals plus one review session was negotiated with Mr B. In fact only six sessions including the review took place. Two aims of therapy were discussed:

- to give awareness of Mr B's consistent state of anxiety and to attempt to reduce this, potentially leading to alleviation of the laryngospasm;
- to give some vocal and personal control to the patient, possibly for the first time. This would be achieved mainly by hypnotherapy techniques but these would, on occasion, be combined with traditional speech and language therapy techniques also delivered in the hypnotic state. Although such techniques had been used previously, the author, in agreement with Abudarham (1991), believed that by offering them in hypnosis, their impact upon the patient would be maximised and anxiety associated with such a conscious delivery would be minimised. Mr B was taught relaxation techniques through hetero- and autohypnosis and was further instructed in the visualisation of his malfunctioning and subsequently appropriately functioning laryngeal musculature. Traditional techniques of slowed and lower tonal speech were taught in hypnosis, aimed at maintaining a relaxed voice, as the higher the tone the more tense the musculature tends to become, and creating belief that some form of spasm control was possible. Other hypnotic techniques were utilised to aid in carrying over skills to everyday situations and to maintain them there.

Hypnotherapeutic interventions

Session 1

On arrival, Mr B was extremely tense, as revealed in his hand wringing and stiff posture whilst perched on the edge of the seat. He had come expecting to be hypnotised and had some preconceived notions about hypnotherapy, mainly as a result of watching stage hypnosis on the television. The first part of the session was therefore spent providing a description of clinical hypnosis in terms of:

- the mind to body connection;
- the vulnerability of the larynx to emotion;
- the conscious and subconscious mind;
- fears and their remediation regarding the forthcoming treatment (Waxman 1989).

The idea of relaxation was introduced and its concept reinforced by asking him to tense up his body very tightly and then to relax it and experience the poignant comparison. He naturally closed his eyes as he did this and then followed instructions to breathe in through his nose and out through his mouth, keeping the outward breath steady. Visualisation of bubble blowing was used to ensure this breath control. Suggestions were then made about progressive relaxation of the body from the top of the head to the tip of the toes alongside further suggestions of limb heaviness and of sinking into the cushions. Mr B displayed a slowing and deepening of breathing, a facial pallor and rapid eye movements during this activity, indicative of an altered state of awareness (Waxman 1989) and so it was suggested to him that he could relax himself in this way at home over the following week. The instructions for achieving this were repeated along with a five-to-one count alerting procedure. On alerting, his ability to utilise these newly taught skills was checked prior to his leaving. A good rapport had been established, evidence of a good trance subject seen and some basic relaxation skills taught. A recording of vocal quality, both when reading a given passage and in natural conversation, was taken before and after hypnotherapy.

Session 2

Mr B arrived in a somewhat anxious state as the morning's post had included an interview date for four weeks hence for a permanent position with a company, which he was desperate to achieve. Imagery for a special place was consciously discussed, which entailed a gentle ski slope down to a snowy mountain scene. At this point a biofeedback machine was used to provide an auditory representation of the anxiety and in order to be able to give the patient further awareness of how it feels to be anxious as opposed to being relaxed. Due to the anxiety, an eye-roll technique (Spiegel 1976) was used to obtain eye closure followed by an induction and deepening routine comprising progressive bodily relaxation and hand levitation (Erikson 1923). The biofeedback machine was left running during these procedures, allowing further monitoring of progressive relaxation for both patient and therapist. The session was recorded with Mr B's permission so that the auditory clarification could be reinforced after hypnosis. Mr B's subconscious mind was addressed and an ideomotor response set up in order to clarify when he felt that he had achieved a deep state of relaxation. From here, the snowball down a mountain (Gibbons 1979) ego strengthening technique was adapted in order to utilise visual, auditory and kinaesthetic modalities. It was

pointed out that Mr B no longer had to be the victim. These suggestions were coupled with those of increasing depth of trance and
acquisition of hypnotic skills. It was then suggested that Mr B
breathe in all these good positive feelings and find the very essence of
his being, which had always been there but had not been accessible
until now. Mr B was advised that he could bring as many of these
feelings, which were now well installed inside his body, back with him
in order to nurture him in the weeks to come. Post-hypnotic suggestions were added, indicating that, with each utilisation of the routine,
the following would be realised: increasing strength of ego-enhanc-
ing suggestions; increasing relaxation experienced and depth of
trance; reduction in time needed to achieve trance.

Mr B was then encouraged to find his chairlift back up the slope
from where he could ski home. A further reminder was given to him
of his ability to return to the special place whenever it was needed.
The patient was alerted using a five-to-one count from where the
acquisition of the routine was checked for use in autohypnosis. Mr B
reported having a wonderful experience and now knew that he had
never actually realised what relaxation was until now. The concept
was further reinforced when the biofeedback monitor was played
back to him. Recordings of vocal quality again took place as
described.

Session 3

On arrival, Mr B reported feeling 'so wonderfully relaxed during
the week' to the extent that he felt the quality of his voice had
improved. He had been practising the self-hypnotic routine every
other day and reported feeling as if a weight had been removed
from his shoulders. Now that the experience of generalised relaxation had been achieved, it was considered necessary to focus these
skills more specifically on to the area responsible for the spasm itself,
the laryngeal musculature. To this end, prior to hypnosis, Mr B, was
shown a simplified picture of the main laryngeal musculature and a
discussion followed about the muscles' attachment to the vocal
cords and their role as a pooling point for excessive bodily tension.
This was reinforced via the example of laryngeal pain, commonly
experienced prior to the onset of tears. The use of hypnotic techniques, such as those given for locating and eradicating tensions,
was therefore also reinforced. Induction and deepening proceedings
were used as described except that in this instance the Spiegel eye-
roll technique (1976) was not needed as the patient felt relaxed
enough just to close his eyes. The ideomotor response taught

previously was again used by Mr B to indicate when trance was deep. At this point metaphor was used to incorporate visualisation of the musculature into therapy. For example, 'I had a patient who had a similar kind of voice to yours and he found it really useful to visualise the muscles of his larynx completely relaxing so that his vocal cords could begin to work regularly and smoothly.' To this end, the idea of a magical spray was utilised. Mr B was to visualise himself spraying his cords once his muscles were relaxed with a magic spray. This would cover them with a special water that would seep in, rendering them moist and flexible. The connection was again suggested between thought and the realisation of physical body changes in order to reinforce this, and the examples of blushing and sexual arousal were given.

Once this had been achieved as indicated by ideomotor response, Mr B was taught traditional techniques of slowed speech (Goldiamond 1965), breath control and gliding of phonological sounds, plus the realisation of a slightly lower vocal tone.

Mr B was reminded of his newly learned traditional therapy and specific visualisation techniques along with the ego-strengthening benefits of frequently visiting his special mountain place. Prior to alerting, post-hypnotic suggestions were then made including those originally given in session one, plus suggestions of increased normality of vocal cord movements in association with relaxed laryngeal musculature with each self-hypnotic attempt. Recordings of vocal quality were again taken.

Session 4

The planning for this session had included commencing exploratory techniques, notably the affect bridge method of age regression (Watkins 1971), as it was felt that much of Mr B's current vocal behaviour was likely to be the result of emotions experienced and subsequent behaviour patterns set up in childhood. The case history certainly seemed to indicate the possibility of this. It was anticipated that ego state therapy (Berne 1967) could potentially be used in order to utilise today's wisdom to reconstruct persistent childhood thinking patterns. However Mr B arrived looking extremely relaxed and happy. He had been using both his autohypnotic routine and traditional methods frequently and reported that two work colleagues had commented on the improved sound of his voice. Interestingly, his immediate family had not done so. He also reported feeling 'So good and relaxed, almost like a new person.' He had been out to the pub with one of his colleagues over the past week, something he had never dared to do previously. To the subjective ear there did seem to be a reduction of vocal tremor and possibly a reduction in frequency of laryngospasm.

As improvements were being seen and as Mr B's job interview was due to take place the following week, and there was new motivation for this, it was jointly decided to abandon these techniques for the time being in order to concentrate on the interview. Induction and deepening took place as described and the technique of age progression was implemented during which Mr B was asked to use his visual, auditory and kinaesthetic channels to experience the forthcoming interview and to rehearse effective coping in the form of deep relaxation with subsequent laryngospasm release. This technique included visualising himself sitting in front of the interviewing panel in a very relaxed state, maintaining eye contact with each panel member as he calmly answered their questions, using his traditional techniques as appropriate. Prior to continuing, his subconscious mind was specifically concerned with whether use of these techniques in this situation was actually going to be workable – whether there were any underlying reasons why the techniques could not be implemented, perhaps reasons of secondary gain. The reply was that there were not, and so the coping strategies generated were anchored (Bandler and Grindler 1979) using a gentle squeeze to the right knee as the trigger stimulus, an action which Mr B felt he could carry out surreptitiously in the interview.

After alerting, the next session was planned for a week after the interview. Mr B was hoping that it would be his last but that he could come back if he needed to. The author felt slightly concerned by this because of the speed with which the patient seemed to have been transformed.

Session 5

Mr B arrived with the news that he had been shortlisted as a result of the interview. It had been a stressful situation for him but the techniques had provided him with calmness and confidence. He further reported that he had been astounded at how much of his life he must have spent in a tense state and was extremely grateful for the help given. The vocal quality appeared to have maintained its improvement, although still could not be classified as falling within normal limits.

A straightforward induction and deepening routine was administered followed by the special place imagery where ego strengthening suggestions and post-hypnotic suggestions of further control, self-confidence, relaxation and reduction in laryngospasm were made.

Mr B reported that he was happy to leave it at that for the time being and so another therapy appointment, although planned, was not made. A review appointment was made for two months hence.

Review session

Prior to the date of this session, Mr B contacted me to say that he could not make the agreed time and he didn't actually feel he needed to come anyway. Although he had not been successful with getting a new job, he regularly practised his techniques as part of a daily schedule and was feeling better about himself than he had ever done before. He was now socialising a lot more and had joined a club attached to a ski slope near his home. His voice and general demeanour still sounded more relaxed with a reduction in the tremor, and there was less breathiness and a marginal reduction in pitch and laryngospasm. He asked if he could be seen again if he needed further help. This was agreed and the patient was discharged.

Discussion

The outcome of this study is positive and indicates that inclusion of hypnotherapy in the treatment of spastic dysphonia of indeterminate origin is of significance because of findings indicating alleviation in the following areas:

Vocal pitch

This was found to be slightly lower after therapy. Reasons for this can only be speculated to be either the result of generalised hypnotic relaxation techniques taught and/or the utilisation of traditional techniques, delivered in hypnosis for heightened impact and tension-reduction purposes.

Breath control

This was arguably due to the generalised hypnotic relaxation techniques used or the multi-modality imagery included of normal respiratory and phonatory mechanisms.

The number of laryngospasms per 10-word sentence.

Improvement seen was marginal and mainly located after session three within natural conversation. Again, we can only speculate that reasons for this improvement might be due to a combination of traditional slowed speech methods delivered in hypnosis, hypnotic imagery involvement and hypnotic relaxation techniques.

Vocal tremor

This was an interesting finding as this area was not directly addressed, but one can surmise that it is another positive by-product of the hypnotic relaxation techniques and the imagery of appropriately functioning vocal apparatus included in these techniques.

Tension

Probably the most dramatic finding of the study, verified by the biofeedback results and reflected in a very swift improvement in quality of life experienced by the patient, notably in the areas of confidence, control and newly found socialisation.

Conclusion

The outcome of the study revealed improvements in a number of different vocal parameters associated with this disorder. Although only relatively marginal, together they proved significant enough to gain positive comments from colleagues. A significant finding was in the seemingly revolutionised effect on lifestyle and ego that the techniques used seemed to bring to the patient in a much shorter time period than traditionally would have been expected. It seems slightly strange that the patient made a firm decision to terminate therapy before the offered therapy block was completed and when further personal and vocal improvements might have been possible. One can only speculate that perhaps the present changes were all that could be accommodated at the present time or that the disorder was associated with some form of secondary gain that remained valuable to the patient.

Following on from this report, it seems essential that clinical trials are carried out in order to compare the effectiveness of hypnotherapeutic techniques used when not combined with traditional speech and language therapy and, indeed, to attempt to provide firm evidence for the argument that the impact of such techniques is heightened when delivered in hypnosis. It also seems imperative to continually follow up such patients to determine whether the benefits are long term or whether future appointments are indicated to provide 'top up' sessions.

The patient's report

During the final telephone call Mr B was asked to comment upon his experiences of the hypnotic intervention. He replied that it had made him feel 'so good and so relaxed'. He added that he felt his voice had improved and he was so much happier with his life and doing so much more than ever before.

Summary

Mr B was referred for treatment of an unusual vocal disorder labelled as spastic dysphonia of indeterminate origin. He had received eight sessions of traditional speech and language therapy previously at another hospital without any improvement being seen. A detailed case history was administered along with traditional speech and language therapy and hypnotherapy assessments. Six treatment sessions plus a review were originally offered with only five actually taken up by the patient. Techniques used involved hypnotherapy as a means of experiencing deep relaxation, ego strengthening, visualisation, autohypnosis and the transfer of skills to the everyday environment. Regressive exploratory techniques were planned but in the event not utilised due to time taken up teaching the concept of relaxation to the patient, and the positive results achieved at an earlier stage than anticipated. More traditional speech and language therapy techniques were also delivered whilst in trance, due to the belief that susceptibility to them and action upon them would be heightened under these circumstances.

On reassessment after therapy, results showed marginal but significant improvement in the overall severity of the dysphonia, with a vast improvement in self-confidence, life control, socialisation and attitude towards the disorder, all reflected in changes and new events within the patient's life.

Hypnotic techniques used in the case reports

The 'is it possible?' protocol (Margolin et al. 1992)

This is an assessment of client susceptibility to hypnosis. The patient is lightly hypnotised and questions are asked: 'Is it possible for you to feel yourself sinking down into the chair?' 'Is it possible for you to be aware of the space within your mouth?' The protocol is delivered in order to establish the client's most effective sensory channel for hypnotic induction and therapy.

Visualisation techniques

These are generally used in hypnotherapy as induction, deepening and therapy techniques. The connection between mind and body seems to be very strong in most people. We know in our own bodies that if we think calm, peaceful thoughts then our bodies respond in a calm way, our breathing slows down, as do our movements, whereas when we think of everything we have to do, our breathing rate soars, we run around, we get physical manifestations of headaches and skin rashes in the short term and who knows what in the long term. So by visualising scenes or indeed perhaps feared events, we can learn to control our fear and calm ourselves down. A colour might be ascribed to a client's tension and then be observed by the client as it is exhaled away.

Ego strengthening

This includes suggestion delivered in hypnosis aimed at enhancing the patient's confidence, self image and sense of wellbeing. It might also include visualisation techniques. An example being to suggest to children that they are eating some magic biscuits, the ingredients of which contain all the good things that have happened in his or her life. Ego strengthening may also be delivered within post-hypnotic suggestions.

Post-hypnotic suggestion

Post-hypnotic suggestion is delivered in hypnosis. It suggests to the client that the current beneficial effects of therapy can carry over into the client's everyday life. Generally suggestions take the form of 'whenever/as soon as you do/think/feel x you will immediately do/think/feel y'.

Anchoring (Bandler and Grindler 1979)

According to Lankton (1980) this is 'any stimulus that evokes a consistent response pattern from a person'. A positive anchor may be attained by asking the client to imagine a situation when he experienced the desired positive feelings and inner strengths to cope with the problem he has. The therapist then touches the client on the knee or wrist and this place then becomes an anchor for the production of those positive feelings when the client requires them.

The Creative imagination scale (Barber and Wilson 1978)

This is an assessment of client hypnotic susceptibility and consists of 10 items that are read aloud to the client who sits relaxing in a chair with his eyes closed. The 10 items are scored by the patient on a 0–4 scale. It is explained to the patient that the purpose of the test is merely to discover what kind of things the patient finds it easy to imagine and then of course the results are used in subsequent induction and therapy.

Self-/autohypnosis

Self-induction and alerting procedures are often taught to the patient in order for him or her to practise deep relaxation at home. Although there is little firm evidence on this subject, experience suggests that the more one uses these techniques, the more deeply and swiftly one is able to relax and the more this relaxed state seems to knock on into other areas of the patient's life.

The Spiegel eye-roll technique (Spiegel 1976)

This is an induction technique used when patients are finding eye closure difficult. The patient is encouraged to roll his or her eyeballs backwards and then to slowly close his lids over them. From here, it is suggested that he lower his eyes downwards in his own time and experience the associated feeling of eye relaxation.

The Affect bridge technique (Watkins 1971)

This is an exploratory technique where it is suggested that the patient regress to the very first occasion when the emotion connected to the current problem was initially experienced, for example a feeling of extreme anger. The patient is then encouraged to focus on this feeling and allow it to become more intense. Imagery used to attain this is usually that of the patient going across a bridge or going down a road surrounded by mist. Once attained, the emotion experienced can be managed therapeutically.

Ego state therapy

This is a technique used to help resolve suspected specific childhood trauma and is based upon the ideas of Berne (1967), who believed there to be three ego states within each client: the child ego, the parent ego and the adult ego. The Patient is initially regressed to the specific traumatic incident and abreaction is allowed to occur. It is then suggested that the adult ego state, with its wisdom gained over time since the incident, go back in time to the child ego state and give it the comfort and reassurance to help it cope with and resolve the trauma.

Age progression

In this technique, it is suggested that the patient is moving forward in time to a visualised future situation. The patient is then encouraged to rehearse a scenario where he or she is coping without difficulty with the new situation. This seems to be a powerful technique for helping patients to cope with the situation in reality.

Chapter 9
Inside the therapeutic relationship

CELIA LEVY AND A CLIENT

Introduction – our backgrounds – maps and models of counselling – our current approaches to counselling – establishing the working alliance – the story of the relationship – final reflections.

Introduction

This chapter tells the story of a counselling relationship that involved a client and myself. The aim is to share aspects of our work, which lasted for 36 sessions spread over one academic year. We have both written about our experiences of the relationship in order to highlight our separate and joint struggles to make contact, reach understanding and grow. To help the reader, the counsellor's story will be told with a regular typeface and the client's will be told in italics. The focus of this chapter will be on the therapeutic relationship and an exploration of how this relationship was understood by us both during our work together.

Our backgrounds

I have stammered ever since I can remember and have always wanted to get rid of it. To this end, I contacted speech therapists at the ages of seven, 16, 18 and 22. All these attempts were unsuccessful and, indeed, the last therapist advised me against seeing a psychologist and to take Valium – something I tried – but it failed. At this point, I gave up on speech therapy and got into alternative practices: yoga breathing, transcendental meditation and others, all of which failed.

Things only changed when I met a speech therapist who taught me the concept of acceptance: stammering more fluently. She introduced me to the works of Van

Riper (1973) and Sheehan (1975). I had some individual and group therapy with her, but always found progress very hard, getting very upset and angry. I had my first experience of counselling with a student who was trying to get me to recognise how I felt about a religious cult I had been in, not what I thought about it. It was a struggle, but I eventually said I felt it was a load of bullshit and felt immediately better! This gave me an inkling of the benefits of counselling.

My therapist felt I might be depressed and wanted me to see a psychotherapist. Initially, I had private treatment at a local hospital. I always wanted individual treatment by somebody with a knowledge of stammering, but this was never available. I also had group therapy, which I didn't find useful, and drama therapy, which was more interesting, but never enough. I had intensive group therapy, which was hard going. My stammering was never mentioned. The therapy I enjoyed the most was art therapy, where I had the realisation that I could communicate emotionally and my stammering was not part of the equation.

I then pursued psychotherapy on the NHS. I had short-term behaviour therapy and cognitive therapy, but only made any real progress when I had short-term psychodynamic counselling. I experienced tremendous amounts of grief about my life and relationships and a sense of failure in my career. I also had an inkling of the importance of the relationship with the counsellor and found that quite challenging. I had a wonderfully supportive GP who helped me face my issues of depression and low self-esteem.

I had made progress in this time after joining the Association for Stammerers (now the British Stammering Association). I made a great leap when I eventually accepted the challenge of a professional career for the first time. However, I found work very stressful: I was forever irritable and exhausted. Ironically, it was only when I had forced myself through all this that I was able to afford counselling at The City Lit with Celia Levy. My self-esteem was up to it and the time was right.

I am a South African qualified speech and hearing therapist. During my training, I became specially interested in the psychological implications of stammering and always knew that I would end up working in this area. Like my client, the ideas of Van Riper (1973) and Sheehan (1975) made great sense to me, and so it was quite a shock to my system when I arrived in the United Kingdom in 1977 to find the approach to stammering therapy was prolonged speech. Fortunately, I was lucky enough to find work at The City Lit (an adult education institute in London) where the open exploration of ideas enabled me to test out and confirm for myself that block modification was indeed the approach I felt happiest using. Staying in the same context for so many years has allowed me to see at first hand why and how people who stammer relapse, despite good initial results from their therapy.

I became interested in training in counselling in order to be a better speech therapist. I started learning about personal construct psychology (Kelly 1955) and, at first, felt that this held all the answers for me. The approach was very different from that of speech therapy but there were enough similarities to create a useful bridge between the two. Both approaches relied heavily on thinking and behaviour, and so I discovered I could expand my approach to stammering without too much inner conflict.

It was when I became more interested in what the humanistic approach to counselling had to offer that my inner turmoil began. I put aside the diagnostic models and began to be with clients in a different way. Now I had no pieces of paper to hide behind, no grids or experiments: it was just the client and I in the room. Finding a humanistic supervisor supported me through the transition I was making and, bit by bit, I realised I could no longer combine the roles of speech therapist and counsellor. I had to choose and I chose counselling. Luckily, The City Lit was able to cope with my self-appointed change in career and the rest is now history!

I met my client at a stage when I had crossed the divide between speech therapy and counselling and called myself a counsellor. The fact that I had specialist knowledge of stammering was very important to him.

Maps and models of counselling

As a speech therapist, I was taught to diagnose the communication disorder and then to plan therapy on the basis of current beliefs about what worked with that particular disorder. This led to a fragmented approach to clients: a more psychological approach for stammering, psycholinguistics for developmental language delays, particular skills and techniques for voice disorders and so forth. I now understand that this approach was focused primarily on the disorder and secondarily on the person. In counselling, this way of working is known as technical eclecticism and is an approach that is entirely driven by results. Technical eclecticists seek to improve our ability to select the best treatment for the person and his or her problem, and the approach chosen tends to be based on research that shows what has worked with similar problems in the past.

I have long struggled with this approach to stammering. Over the years, different speech techniques have replaced others and I have always had an uneasy belief that all of them work more-or-less well. I used to wonder how important technique was. Then, when I studied personal construct therapy, I was invited to ask myself why I did what I did, and to develop a coherent theoretical basis for my work. At last, I began to clarify what my core beliefs about people and therapy were as a basis for choosing what to do in therapy. At last, I was learning an approach to the person and not merely techniques to use on their problems.

This way of thinking about therapy is known as philosophical or theoretical integration. What is not implied is that I have to seek out the 'best' theory and adhere to a single approach. Integration implies that a new approach is created out of combining aspects of different approaches in creative ways. Thus, eclecticism provides a smorgasbord approach to therapy whereas integration creates new dishes by combining different ingredients (Norcross and Arkowitz 1992).

One way of approaching integration of different models is to look at the nature of the counselling relationship. As the client and counsellor are always in relationship, this is at the heart of most approaches to counselling. I have evolved a pictorial representation of the different therapeutic relationships and how they relate to each other (see Figure 8.1). The text that follows explains each relationship in more detail.

In order for 'help' to be of use, a *working alliance* needs to be established. Many approaches refer to this in different ways. Some form

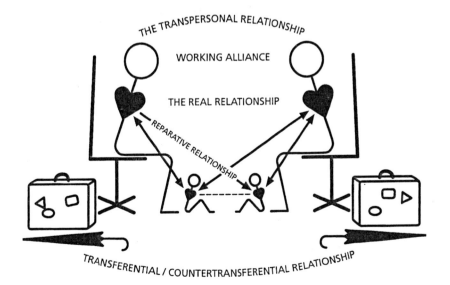

Figure 9.1: The multiplicity of therapeutic relationships.

of contract is usually established that determines the rules of engagement: the main boundaries that have to be maintained. In transactional analysis (Berne 1964) the working alliance is seen as the Adult–Adult agreement. This is where counsellors set out what they do and how they do it and clients choose to work with them or not. Doctors give advice and prescriptions: the patient is required to follow instructions in order to get well. Similarly, speech therapists set up a therapeutic regime that requires cooperation between therapist and patient for it to work. A useful definition of the working alliance is that it is 'the part of the client–psychotherapist relationship that enables the client and therapist to work together even when the patient or client experiences some desires to the contrary' (Clarkson 1995, p. 31).

Second, there is a *transferential/countertransferential relationship*, which is very well described within the psychoanalytic tradition. Freud was not aiming to cure patients, but was rather searching for understanding.

'The transferential/countertransferential relationship is the experience of unconscious wishes and fears transferred on to or into the therapeutic partnership' (Clarkson 1995, p. 62). No relationship is immune to these aspects and transference can positively enable therapy to be therapeutic. For example, faith in the therapist can strengthen the working alliance. Different approaches pay more or less attention to transferential factors. Not to attend to the more overt transferential issues could be very harmful to the process. For example, have you ever felt an overwhelming desire to see a client more often than has been agreed? Has one of your clients ever said anything to you that makes you feel uncomfortable? Knowing more about the dynamics of a relationship can throw light on these unconscious processes.

Third, we have the *reparative/developmentally needed relationship*. This is the intentional provision by the therapist of a corrective or replenishing parental relationship where original parenting was deficient, abusive or overprotective (Clarkson 1995, p. 11). This relationship provides reparenting. Before therapists purposefully work in this way with clients, they need to be aware of the awesome professional and ethical responsibilities they are taking on.

Fourth, there is the *person-to-person relationship*, which is the real relationship as opposed to an object relationship. Buber (1958) wrote about the 'I–thou' relationship. In the humanistic tradition, it is believed that healing takes place through this relationship. Both client and therapist exist in a kind of mutuality in the here and now.

The real person of the therapist cannot be excluded from the therapeutic encounter as a major psychotherapeutic modality. As much as the psychoanalyst tries to present a blank screen to attract the transferential reactions of the client, that therapist is also a real person in the encounter and will share the same human frailties as the client.

For Rogers (1951, 1967), the establishment of a relationship of genuineness, respect and empathy became the cornerstone for facilitating human growth and development. This relationship is honoured by truthfulness and authenticity. The relationship becomes a partnership.

Finally, the *transpersonal relationship* is the timeless facet of the psychotherapeutic relationship, which is more difficult to describe, but refers to the spiritual dimension of the healing relationship. This aspect acknowledges qualities that presently transcend the limits of our understanding. Many therapists cannot account for unaccountable and incomprehensible outcomes in therapy except through this seemingly mystical experience.

> Implied is a letting go of skills, of knowledge, of experience, of preconceptions, even of the desire to heal, to be present. It is essentially allowing 'passivity' and receptiveness for which preparation is always inadequate. But paradoxically, you have to be full in order to be empty. It cannot be made to happen, it can only be encouraged in the same way that the inspirational muse of creativity cannot be forced, but needs to have the ground prepared or seized in the serendipitous moment of readiness. What can be prepared are the conditions conducive to the spontaneous or spiritual act. (Clarkson 1995, p. 20.)

These five relationships are available as potential avenues for constructive use. To use them knowingly and purposefully is to bring a sense of responsibility to bear on therapeutic work. Being aware of the different relationships may be one of the most important ways of integrating different therapeutic approaches. This map can also provide a structure for maintaining boundaries between different approaches to counselling. For example, if therapists do not feel trained to work with one or more of the relationships described above, they will be more able to set limits on their work and act within their ethical responsibilities.

In my experience, to work outside the working alliance requires consistent use of supervision because the potential for entanglement or self-deception about what is truly going on is obvious. Another pair of eyes with supervision skills is most certainly required.

Our current approaches to counselling

I had done a lot of reading over the years and had been most influenced by the work of Joseph Sheehan (1975) and his avoidance reduction therapy. I knew I avoided a lot and therefore would have a hard time in therapy. I became fascinated by his five levels of avoidance: word, situation, emotion, relationship and ego-protective. His view was that speech therapy would only address the first two, whereas psychotherapy would be needed for the last three. He thought the ideal therapist for a person who stammers should be a speech therapist and psychotherapist. I became convinced that this was what I wanted as no one else had seemed to understand and explain my own stammering better than Sheehan. I had also become fascinated by my childhood experiences and how they affected me and had developed an interest in transactional analysis (Berne 1964).

I view myself primarily as a humanistic counsellor, influenced by the person-centred approach of Carl Rogers (1951, 1961, 1980) and existentialists such as Yalom (1980). It has been said that the person-centred approach is particularly light on theory, but those who practise it are in no doubt that it is one of the most rigorous and demanding approaches.

The person-centred model has as its central concern the experience of the individual human being and the importance of his or her subjective reality. Clients take responsibility for their own lives and learn to trust their inner resources (Mearns and Thorne 1988). The existentialist belief that we can fulfil our potential is fundamentally important to me.

Growth in counselling is facilitated by the quality of the relationship between counsellor and client. The counsellor's use of self is at the heart of this approach. The counsellor attempts to create a climate for growth by demonstrating the core conditions in her way of being with the client. The first of these conditions is congruence or genuineness: the desire and ability to be truly oneself. Being real within the counselling relationship involves taking the risk of showing my real self, being willing to be seen as I am, as an equal and not as an expert. Secondly, unconditional positive regard is an attitude of total acceptance of the client as he is at this time. It implies that no judgements of the client's way of being will impede the client from being able to bring difficult aspects of himself or herself into the open. Perhaps this core condition inspires trust. The third element is empathy, a process of being able to step into the client's shoes and accurately feel and sense what the client is experiencing.

Over the years, I have found myself increasingly drawn towards trying to understand some of the unconscious elements of the counselling relationship. I have had only minimal training in psychodynamic theory, but the key concepts of transference and counter-transference have always made sense to me.

Transference reactions arise out of the fact that we tend to view important relationships in the present through templates developed in our earliest relationships (Kahn 1991). Transference, as a process, is not limited to therapy, but is present to a greater or lesser extent in all relationships. In counselling, working with transference reactions provides useful material for gaining an understanding of, and bringing into awareness, how clients react to the counsellor in the light of their earliest relationships.

Countertransference refers to the counsellor's reactions to the client. Kahn (1991) refers to two hidden dramas being played out in the therapeutic relationship: that of the client and that of the therapist. It is expected that therapists should have resolved most issues in their lives but it is not possible to achieve a state of perfection. Countertransference reactions can be useful in throwing light on what might be going on for the client. If I feel very maternal towards a client, could this arise from the way in which the client relates to me? If the client is flattering, do I feel better about myself? Are my responses to this client different from my responses to other clients or people in general? What can I learn from my own reactions here and now?

In my work, I aim to be very real and present in the counselling relationship as a humanistic practitioner. I do not go out of my way to cultivate transference reactions by presenting the client with a blank screen as a psychodynamic practitioner would. However, being mindful of transferential issues that arise and drawing on these to make sense of the client's experiences is helpful.

With reference to Figure 8.1, my work involves the explicit use of three relationships: the working alliance, the real relationship and the transferential/countertransferential relationship. It is possible that my counselling work has reparative elements within in it, but, because my work is time-limited, I do not aim to take on reparenting as a therapeutic task. The mysterious transpersonal relationship may also arise with certain clients. I certainly have experienced an intuitive sense of knowing and a sense of contact beyond words with these clients.

Philosophical integration of different models involves arriving at a new approach that is greater than the sum of the parts. Although not my own term, I have come to call my approach to counselling 'dynamic humanism'.

Establishing the working alliance

Before a client and counsellor ever meet, expectations are likely to influence their first encounter. Both the client and the therapist will have prepared for their meeting. Their prior knowledge of each other will affect the relationship that follows.

Let me tell you what was in my mind before I ever met my client for our first counselling session. A City Lit colleague referred him to me for counselling in July 1995. I noticed a feeling of surprise in myself. Ever since he had moved to the South East I had been expecting this moment. Why had he not contacted me directly? We had already met previously when he lived in the North West. At that stage, he had wanted to work with me, but I had suggested that he continue to work with a local speech therapist, taking it upon myself to decide that weekly journeys to London would be very demanding. I didn't admit to myself or to him that I feared the pressure of his high expectations of me.

In September we met to discuss working together. I was somewhat nervous, wondering whether or not he now had a more realistic view of counselling and what I could offer him. I knew he would have read what I had written on stammering and since I had written my last piece on the subject (Hayhow and Levy 1989) I had changed considerably. What would he think of my current approach to counselling?

He arrived early, also looking anxious. He chose to sit near the door. Later he told me that he needed an escape route in case he wanted to leave the room suddenly. I have learned that how people arrive and leave sessions is very important (Hawkins and Shohet 1989). He established a routine of putting down his briefcase and taking off his jacket and jumper. I sensed he needed a ritual as a way of entering my space. He seldom spoke as he prepared himself. Then he would sit down and establish eye contact with me. I would usually remain silent and wait for him to begin. Often these moments were intense and provocative. More often than not, I would smile and acknowledge his presence, but usually I would not speak. Eventually he would begin.

Right at our first meeting I mentioned our prior contact and our relationship through the British Stammering Association. Did this make a difference to him? Was there anything we needed to get out of the way in order to begin this new phase in our relationship? He looked surprised and asked if he was correct in assuming that every-thing we discussed would be confidential. I hardly had time to nod before he went on: he had prepared what he wanted to talk about. This was not the time to discuss our relationship.

I had always wanted the 'best therapist' for myself and did consider this was Celia. I was in awe of her and she did make me feel a little uncomfortable, espe-cially when she mentioned this at the start. I was very pleased she could give me a year of therapy, but disappointed it could not be more. She handled the issues of payment very well.

He told me a bit about his life. He raised huge questions about many choices he had made in his life. It was as if he didn't trust that any decision he had made was for the right reasons. He described himself as a failure. I noticed that he used two key words to describe his feel-ings: 'shocked' and 'upset'. Other than this, he talked about himself in a strongly analytical and cognitive way.

Near the end of the session, I offered him time to ask me any questions. He wanted to know about results, methods. I explained that my counselling was based on the person-centred approach: that I had no answers, but trusted that we could find them together. I also mentioned that our relationship would be important to the process and that we would talk about it frequently. He said he felt more able to take responsibility for himself.

Supervision issues

At the end of our first session, I felt many things, but most of all anxious about agreeing to work together. I still felt as if I was going to be on trial. Would I play to this? Did I need him to admire my work? I wondered even then if the one year of counselling on offer was going to be sufficient. Should I take him on? How was I going to deal with his anger that I sensed was seething below the surface? One superficial similarity threw up a huge difference between us: we would both be the same age at our next birthday and yet we saw ourselves so differently. Would I be able to understand him and truly empathise with him? I realised that I would have to open up some very scary places in myself if I was going to be able to stay with his feelings of despair and failure. Not to do so would mean ending up behaving towards him like his father had: judging him, telling him to pull himself together and get on with life. This had not worked for him. Our relationship was going to have to be different.

I spent much of my next supervision session looking at this first meeting. I had just started working with a new supervisor and I think many of the parallel processes went missing because of it. Looking back, I think I behaved in supervision in much the same way that my client behaved with me. I wanted an answer from my supervisor: should I work with him or not? I didn't want to explore my feelings about the relationship. I noticed myself resisting facing what was going on within me. However, I decided to take him on and felt supported enough to know that I would have the necessary backup to help me cope with the despair that I was sure would be triggered by this work.

The story of the relationship

A positive transference can be helpful to the work (Jacobs 1988). This client wanted to work with me and approached his counselling with commitment. I was very aware that his expectations and hopes might exceed what was possible, and therefore decided that one of the ways in which I might usefully approach our work together would be to play an ordinary role. I would not be the expert; I would not have the answers. I needed to be watchful of his need to cast me in a role where I carried responsibility for him.

The most shocking thing for me was to realise that I was in an equal partnership and she was not going to tell me what to do. It took a while to get used to this: I can see the need in me for a guru. This did wonders for my self-esteem, as did the person-centred approach of empathy, congruence and unconditional positive regard. I think I had always felt my parents had viewed me as bad and a failure and I had taken this self-image on board. It was a struggle to feel that Celia felt differently about me. I could not handle the positive feelings that I had about her and I couldn't express them verbally. I daren't be angry with her in case she rejected me and that would have been horrible. I was always surprised when she didn't.

A significant moment occurred in our third session. We had spent much time discussing counselling. Again he was asking lots of questions. Then he said that although he had had some therapy, he hadn't 'faced some of the dark areas' of his psyche. Suddenly he asked, 'Will you stay with me, Celia?' I nodded and said 'That seemed like an important question'. His eyes filled with tears and he seemed full of emotion.

He seemed to be asking me if it was safe enough to trust me. Would it be safe enough for him to let go? Would I make the commitment to him to see it through with him? I felt very moved. I felt that I had agreed to work with him in my entirety. I could be truly congruent with him about this. We had connected for the first time: heart to heart. We had begun.

Very early in our work, the client had a 'crisis' at work: he had 'ground to a halt' and gone home. He had not been to work the next day. He explained that he had run away. He described his behaviour as similar to a child having a temper tantrum. There was something different about his way of talking to me, as if he was being quite defiant. I certainly felt as if he was communicating from a childlike place. My question to myself was how to be in relation to him. I sensed that he longed for me to sweep him up and tell him that he never had to go back to work ever again. If he was in child mode, then was I in parent mode? He certainly seemed in need of 'parenting', but the strategy I chose was to acknowledge his longing, but not to meet the need. I had to help him recover his ability to go back to work and face whatever was there. I trusted that he had the capacity to do just this, but knew it would be hard. This is what we worked on.

Being aware of both transference and countertransference reactions enabled me to voice what was going on, but not to act on it. I said 'I'm aware that you want to run away, and perhaps are even asking me for permission to do so. I can feel the depth of your feeling about this. At the same time, I know that you know that this is not possible. So, I'm wondering how we can work together to find a way for you to get back to work?'

That session ended with him in tears. I felt very sad, but relieved as well. He said that he felt able to go to work the next day and did. What he had been able to do was to share very deep feelings of sadness, helplessness and grief. He was not so alone.

Another theme, already alluded to, was his need to have a guru in his life. I was aware that I could and perhaps already had taken on this role. It felt important not to collude with his need for me to be an expert. Kohut (in Kahn 1991) asserts that all children have a need to idealise and to believe that at least one parent is powerful and knowledgeable. This parent will help the child to deal with both an internal and external world that is frightening or threatening in some way.

Imagine a child growing up stammering. The importance of parental help in resolving some of the complex feelings associated with communication difficulties cannot be underestimated. What if the parents are afraid that stammering is their fault and that they have somehow failed their child? What if stammering is a problem they cannot resolve and somehow expect the child to sort things out for himself? I imagine that something along these lines happened in my client's family. His own sense of failure and his need for expertise outside himself was very deep rooted. Whenever anyone slipped into the role of expert in his life, knowingly or unknowingly, a recurring pattern of idealisation followed by failure would occur.

In his relationship with me, as in his relationship to other therapies and therapists, he had an intense longing for an expert, for a 'powerful parent' who would resolve his problems. The challenge of my approach to the counselling relationship was enormous, but of vital importance. His expertise on himself and ability to decide for himself how to tackle things was the only way forward. This meant that I had to frustrate his need for answers, and tolerate a state of 'not knowing' myself. Throughout our work, this was the aspect of our work that was the most difficult for me. I feel sure that I slipped into the role of 'expert' over and over again. My own conflict was between my role as speech therapist and my role as counsellor. As a speech therapist, rightly or wrongly, I had learned to behave more like an expert than in my role as counsellor. My client soon found ways of pushing those old buttons and I would fall into the trap and tell him what I thought. This would lead to short-term gratification and long-term disillusionment.

Looking back at my notes, I see that I wrote 'I sense he needs good mothering, fathering and friendship. By enabling him to feel his feelings, I am threatening his "fortress". I feel quite trapped, which seems to mirror how he feels. For him to let go he needs to trust me. He wants me to be clever, an expert, but perhaps he needs to see me as trustworthy? Maybe then he will begin to work.'

In the next session I encountered what I experienced as his resistance to our work. He told me that he didn't want to blame his parents for anything. He found it so hard to blame them. He thought that having therapy was a sign of weakness on his part. His father had always told him to pull himself together. His mother had wanted him to become a bank clerk, a safe job. He had been taught to aim low by his mother and yet he felt that he would always disappoint his father by not achieving enough.

He was angry with me. I wondered if he sensed that I had expectations of him too and that he didn't want to fail or disappoint me. In talking about his childhood the previous week, he had begun to see his parents differently. He had lost his ability to idealise his father and wanted that back. He needed to see himself as a failure: to take on another view was perhaps very threatening. He was lost and ungrounded.

The following week he told me he thought he felt depressed. He'd read a book on depression (Rowe 1983) that week and decided he could 'have depression'. The particular book he had read emphasised that depression was a choice. He was back to blaming himself.

We spent some time evaluating our work that week as it was the end of the first term. He was very negative. He said he was still struggling with the idea that I was not going to solve his problems for him. I asked him if he felt disappointed: his eyes filled and he started to say something, but couldn't go on. My sense was that he wanted to express anger and stopped himself. It was a difficult place to stop for the Christmas holidays.

Despite being a difficult time to stop for a break, I was very encouraged by his negativity. Was this going to be the beginning of a negative transference? If he saw me as failing him like his parents had done, this might give him the chance of expressing the feelings towards his parents that he never had let himself feel before. The difference would be that I would be willing to hang in there with him and accept him and his negative feelings. Perhaps he would be able to learn to express his anger and know that it would not destroy either him or me.

The next term, we returned to his unspoken feelings. He tried to explain that when he feels something powerfully, he can't think or hear or respond to the world outside himself. We began to discover that he senses rather than feels emotions. He experiences bodily sensations: tingling in the legs, a sense of his head getting larger and lighter, tightness in his neck. Perhaps this might explain his paucity of words to describe feelings. His bodily sensations have meaning for him but are difficult to communicate and not visible on the outside.

In this counselling, I felt I had the opportunity and the time to confront myself as an emotional being and to confront the level of grief I had about myself, my stammer and my sense of failure in life. I cried very hard several times with Celia, and was always fighting it back. Occasionally Celia would voice what she thought I was feeling, and a torrent would burst out. I had to hang on and let myself feel it: but beyond was a larger grief that I could not let myself feel.

We never got to my other main emotion that was anger. I did get angry about a religious cult I had joined when I was younger, a stupid mistake I made in my life. Every therapist I have met has thought I am an angry man, but I find this very hard to accept in myself. One big thing I learnt with Celia is that there are very powerful emotions in me that I have denied and that I have to be ready to experience them. Repressing them has its penalties of depression. Another major surprise was the depth of my anxiety at the thought of not stammering, another major plank of Sheehan's work. I was totally surprised at the amount of hidden anxiety that my stammer may have been protecting me from. To experience strong physical symptoms of anxiety at the thought of being fluent was shocking, frightening and liberating at the same time. At last I had some real understanding of my avoidances. I always felt I was not succeeding in speech therapy and therefore needed psychotherapy to unblock my resistances.

I had wonderful moments in therapy, usually after I had faced something upsetting, where I felt calm and relaxed, my speech slowed down and I stammered more with a lot less tension. I think it is a state of feeling happy while stammering that I had not experienced before. I was always upset, though, because I knew it wouldn't last. However, I got great benefit knowing that I had experienced it and therefore could do so again.

Celia had three views of me that I found hard to come to terms with, which she saw much more easily than me. One was that I was very impatient: I had to work very hard at slowing down but did come to recognise the truth of less haste, more speed. Second, that I was hard on myself: something I still can't accept. Third, that I was perfectionistic: I struggled with this one too, but eventually came to see my idealisation of myself as 'a perfect fighting machine' as laughable.

A major realisation I had during the counselling was that changing something about yourself can be hard. I hadn't really appreciated that before. I had also thought that psychotherapy must be easy because it was for failures; failures were weak people, and therefore the therapy must be easy so they could succeed. I do not think this now. I found my counselling painful and had to face this. I came to respect Celia's honesty and courage and that helped me find my own.

During the second term, our work went into deeper issues and our relationship continued to develop. At the end of one session my client told me rather apologetically that he had read a book on person-centred counselling by Mearns and Thorne (1988). He hadn't been able to tell me the week before and felt bad reading it behind my back, as if he was checking up on me. I had the sense he felt like a naughty child, messing around with grown-up books. Did he expect me to punish him?

In actual fact, I was rather pleased that he had ventured into reading counselling books. Even if he felt 'naughty', his action was a way of honouring the equality we were striving for in our relationship. His right to know what I was doing and why I was doing it would help to redress the imbalance in our relationship. Here, I am commenting on the adult-to-adult relationship, rather than the transferential relationship. This alliance provides the container within which transference reactions can be expressed.

What might he have been re-enacting in our relationship? Had he spied on his parents as a child? Did his parents have secrets? Would knowing my secrets make me lose power? Our time was up and I never did find out.

Half-way through the second term, he arrived angry and upset for his session. Things were going badly at work: he was 'grinding to a halt'. He was angry with me again. He had felt the last few sessions had been very powerful and were going too fast, making things difficult for him. At work, he felt pushed around by stress and what he really wanted to do was escape. However, that would make him feel bad too. For him, work was a way of succeeding in life.

I reflected his ambivalence to him. One part of him wanted to work and that part sounded very grown up. Another part didn't want to work. He felt that part of him was about six or seven years old. This part was linked to his stammering, and avoidance. Suddenly he realised that as a child he had never been allowed to express feelings, most especially anger. His father could not cope with his feelings. I wondered if he was worried that his anger might be too much for me? Very quickly he said 'No!' Was it too much for him? 'Maybe.' Was he protecting himself and/or me? This really was an important question for him. He realised that he could be spending his life protecting people from his negative feelings.

What had transpired in this session was an important way of working in counselling. The client first talks about something going on for him outside in his life. In this case, he mentioned his angry feelings about work. The counsellor then looks to see if these feelings relate to anything in the client–counsellor relationship. The connection was quickly made in our session. The client also felt pushed by me and was angry with me. Then the counsellor invites the client to look at how these here and now feelings might be related to past events. He soon realised how angry he felt with his father but couldn't express the anger in any of the situations in his life, because his father could not cope. Jacobs (1988, p. 104) refers to this process as the 'Triangle of Insight'.

In the next session my client said that he had had a glimpse of the way things might be in the future. He felt he had more space in which to manoeuvre. Part of him wanted to go for it, but a more cautious part of him was frightened. He had a headache over his left brow, which always signalled that things were about to change for the worse. He remembered that his father had always given him contradictory messages: 'say you can, and you will' versus 'you lack moral fibre'. As with so many other conflicts, his response was at a bodily level: his headache symbolised how stuck he could feel.

We discussed the possibility of expressing his feelings openly, rather than through his physical suffering. He was very angry as he realised how he had never been able to express his feelings honestly. This was the first time he had been able to be critical of his parents in a more sustained way. The following week he reported a dream in which he had shouted and physically expressed angry feelings. He had not harmed anyone and had reached a quiet acceptance at the end of the dream. I wondered if he was beginning to allow this split-off part of himself to integrate into his so-called 'good' side.

Over the next few weeks, he reported allowing himself to express a variety of different feelings outside our sessions. It felt as if he was colouring in unused parts of himself. His experiences of deep emotions in sessions also became apparent. In one session he talked about how he had felt about being part of his wife's family, who were passionately connected to each other. When he thought about his own family he saw something bad and pinched. He gestured with his hand, pulling ugly faces as if he could taste something awful and bitter. He realised that his mother had not been able to love him enough. Physical contact with her was minimal. He wondered why he was not seeing his sister much these days.

I commented that he seemed to be talking about female love. When he talked about his wife's family, he described something swirling around him: a kind of female energy. It had a billowing feeling, swirling around him, holding him. He started to have strange feelings in his body now: tingling legs. He jumped up, saying he felt sensations in his head, nausea and headache all at once. He didn't know what it meant, only that we were onto something.

He felt sad that his mother hadn't loved him enough. He didn't want to think of her like that. As soon as he mentioned her, his face started grimacing and he held his hand in a vulture-like position. He looked like he wanted to spit and shudder. We had to bring the session to a close at this point: time was up. How much safer he seemed to feel, and how much more himself he was able to be!

In the last session of the Spring term, my client told me that he and his wife had decided to have a summer holiday, and that they were not going to invite his father to come along. This seemed like a hugely significant event for him: a declaration of boundaries and a valuing of himself and his family.

We spent some time reviewing the term's work. He felt that he related differently to me now. He had retrieved some of the power he had given me by reading four books on counselling this term. He asked me to be more challenging next term and said that he wanted to explore our relationship in more depth. Although he said he felt all right about the break, I caught a look of fright in his eyes as he left that indicated other feelings that were around.

Our final term began on quite a positive note with my client saying that he felt better about himself overall. In his view, he felt that, having tackled feelings, he was now ready to move on to exploring relationships (Sheehan 1975).

We decided to begin by looking at our relationship the next week. He found it very difficult to know how to begin to discuss this: he squirmed in his seat and seemed more agitated than usual. With a bit of prompting, he said that he felt more like himself in our relationship than anywhere else, but could not identify what made this possible. Even so, he still expected me to be an expert and someone he could look up to. He felt very uneasy trying to view our relationship as an equal one. I acknowledged that there were real differences and invited him to say more about how he felt in our relationship.

What struck me very forcibly is that he had only a small vocabulary with which to discuss relationships. I remember reflecting to him that I felt that he saw me more like a robot therapist than as a person. He said that he didn't want to know me as a person, or to think of me as having my own life. He longed for someone who truly understood him. I sensed that he felt that perhaps I did not understand him. He looked upset. I asked him to try to say what he was feeling. He struggled unsuccessfully and suddenly I felt that I could sense what he was feeling. I spoke in the first person: 'I am alone with my stammering. I am frightened and isolated. I need someone to make sense of what I am feeling so that I can understand it myself. I need someone to see the real me, to love me enough so that I can have faith in myself.' He buried his head in his hands and wept. Perhaps he truly experienced his existential separateness at that moment, but, paradoxically, he could feel as well that he was not entirely alone.

The next week brought him to the session feeling rather agitated. He explained that he hadn't wanted to leave at the end of the last session. He had wanted to write to me during the week, but thought he should stick to the boundaries of our sessions, and so didn't. He wanted to apologise for attacking me for not understanding him and then I had demonstrated that I really did understand him. He had felt very touched and moved by our exchange. He was still feeling fragile and uncomfortable.

This was an important development in our relationship. He had felt uncomfortable about what he had said to me, and yet was able to contain his feelings for a week. He had expressed anger and feared it had been destructive, that I might reject him and at the same time was confident enough of our relationship to hold on to his anxiety and talk about it next time.

Over the next few weeks, I was more and more able to express the empathy I felt and it seemed more accurate. He used my under-standing as a way of connecting to some deep feelings of grief and wept copiously in our sessions. He was letting me see him as he experienced himself. I think he felt dazed by our work: I was aware of feeling exhausted at the ends of sessions.

He became almost obsessed with his feelings of anger. He wanted to express anger, and was bitterly disappointed that he could not or would not do so. Sometimes it seemed that his angry hurricane would blow my way but at the last minute he would veer off. I started to become anxious about the fact that we had only a few sessions left. I wondered if he was feeling the same way.

He told me he could not be angry with me because of all the messages he had received from his parents. He was supposed to be civilised, polite, clean, clever, middle class. Being angry means being a yob, working class, not clever. Because he saw me as being sophisticated and clever, he found it hard to be angry with me. He was worried that I would not like the crude, yobbish side of him.

To discover that I might be blocking his anger was difficult and something that I spent time discussing in supervision. My supervisor and I worked out ways he could express his anger without words, and each time I prepared for this, he wanted to talk about something else. It was frustrating for me and for him. I felt that I was failing him. It was useful to explore my countertransference reactions. Some of what was blocking him might have been my fear of anger leading to violence and lack of experience of dealing with it. Not so long ago, I had an experience with a client who had become angry and then violent in the session, and had destroyed some of her own treasured possessions which she had brought to show me. On her exit from my office, she had kicked the door so hard that it had to be rehung. I know I had felt very shaken by this episode, and despite much work on my reactions, I was perhaps not ready yet to invite the open expression of anger in my rather small office.

We now began to discuss the end of our work together. Apart from processing some of the feelings this raised, what did he want to do next? This provoked much anxiety over the next few sessions. About six sessions from the end, he arrived after having a couple of days off work. He was feeling very angry. He was finding it hard to cope with work. Our therapy was ending, and we had not solved anything. He could not afford private psychotherapy. He was feeling frightened and angry. He burst into tears and released some of the pent-up emotion this way. He calmed down and became more at one with himself.

The next week he said that he hadn't wanted to come and see me, and had thought about stopping before our time was up. He was feeling very sorry for himself. Finally, he acknowledged that he didn't want our work to come to an end. This enabled him to commit to coming for the last few sessions.

He missed the third-last session, but came for his second-last session. He felt very sad. We focused on our ending – a forced ending, rather than one coming at a time when it was right to stop working together. He told me that he thought he had engineered moving South especially so that he could see me for counselling. I wondered if he felt disappointed that he was not feeling very good now. Yes, he was disappointed, but he assured me it was not my fault, as usual taking the blame himself.

At our last session, he seemed to be in better shape than he had been for some time. We talked about our work together. He remembered asking me if I would stay with him, and felt that I had. He now felt more equal to me and that he had overcome some of his past issues with me. He realised that he did find it very difficult to talk about our relationship, but had still learned a lot about it. He commented that he felt he could never pull the wool over my eyes. I was a strong woman and he liked that. It stopped him from being flirtatious with me.

At the very end, we said our goodbyes with some of the awkwardness that had been there at the start. Having shared so much at such deep levels along the way, the social level of the goodbye seemed inadequate. He left and I breathed out.

Six months later

At the end of the counselling, I found myself suffering from stress and unable to go to work. My doctor prescribed a course of treatment for my anxiety. After two weeks off work and two weeks holiday, I was ready to go back to work. While I was on holiday I came to realise how stressful I found certain aspects of my life, especially related to my speech. I realised more fully the depth of my upset and how I didn't readily share it with anyone. I was able to do so with my wife for perhaps the first time, and felt stronger for it. I was now able to make a big decision at work about the future direction of my career that I had been struggling with for several years. I felt wonderful after doing this and have been feeling better ever since. I'm sure my counselling played a big part in this as well as the treatment.

After my counselling, I was able to decide to do a course of speech therapy at The City Lit: their two-term group evening course for interiorised stammering. Again, this is something I had unsuccessfully been trying to achieve for several years, and I believe my counselling helped me to do it.

Progress on the course was slow, and I touched on the old emotions of grief and anger. I rode a strong desire to leave when I first had to confront constructing my hierarchy of desensitisation. I also had a very powerful experience at the end of the first term where I got in touch with deep feelings of anger about my stammer and the effect it had had on my life. I was shouting and swearing to the group, but it felt good!

Towards the end of the group, I was able to get back in touch with very power-ful feelings about the ego-protective nature of my stammering (Sheehan's fifth level of avoidance) and the psychological threats to myself in losing it. I have suffered from a 'giant in chains' complex. I have felt for a long time that the reason why I am not more successful is because of my stammer. I feel lost without my stammer: for then I have no excuse not to succeed and I may fail, which I fear. I have recog-nised a very powerful 'childish' voice in me saying: 'I don't want to fail because no one will love me.' Because my imperfect speech was unacceptable to my parents, I have tried to be perfect all my life, and that is an intolerable strain. I have used my stammering as a protection against the threat of failure that success brings. Obvi-ously any progress I make towards controlling my stammering causes psychologi-cal resistances fuelled by these fears of failure. I feel blown apart by the possible truth of Sheehan's premise that accepting your stammering is a hard task, but coming to terms with the problems of fluency can be even harder.

Prior to counselling the only way I could feel good was to tell myself how much more successful I would have been if I didn't stammer. I have always previously resisted getting control of my stammer through speech therapy because I couldn't face my anxieties about failure. I had to shatter the illusion that I would be a different person if I didn't stammer and accept myself as I really am, stammer and all. This is a heady freedom that I am still getting used to. I can be myself. I don't have to pretend I would have been a great success but for my stammer, yet I don't need to let my stammer hold me back.

I feel I have made a great step in speech therapy that I was only able to make after having counselling. I am interested now in developing my assertiveness and being my own man. I want to get to know myself as a man who speaks dysflu-ently. How do I feel? What do I want to do?

Final reflections

Working with this client stretched me beyond what I might have predicted when we started out together. I believe our work took courage and that he demonstrated his bravery and determination throughout the counselling process and beyond. His willingness to share his story stands testimony to his ability to be himself and live in the open. I am deeply grateful to him.

At the end of writing this chapter I feel clearer about the role of counselling in speech therapy. Although it complicated matters in some ways, my knowledge of stammering enabled me to work better as a counsellor with this client. I was not afraid of the enormity of stammering, and could challenge his need to discuss his speech when I felt it might be stopping us exploring other more difficult issues. At other times, I could listen to his feelings about stammering and share my knowledge and experience in this field.

Our work was not smooth and its ending did not bring about a 'cure' or even great happiness. However, what is apparent from his own evaluation of his counselling, is that he is once more on the move, having trusted himself to make important life choices. That he did this outside our relationship is a mark of the success of our work together. His ability to make good use of speech therapy after coun-selling and become more self-accepting illustrates the importance of not choosing one approach above the other, but of having both counselling and speech therapy available as avenues of change for clients with communication difficulties.

My client and I were fellow travellers for a time, and each of us in our own way has continued on our separate journeys. I feel enriched by the time we spent together.

Chapter 10
Andrew: psychoanalytic psychotherapy with an autistic child

GRAHAM SHULMAN

'I would sit . . . listening to the story as though [my father] were one of my story-telling records. In my head I would do the introduction: "this is an original little long-playing record, and I am your storyteller. We are going to begin now to read the story" . . . .'

Donna Williams, *Nobody Nowhere*

Introduction – referral – early history – assessment: initial meeting – assessment individual sessions – therapy – the fourth year of therapy – theoretical background – summary.

Introduction

This chapter is an account of the gradual and precarious develop-ment of self in a boy with mild-to-moderate autism, whom I shall call Andrew. Andrew had just turned four when he started three-times-weekly individual psychoanalytic psychotherapy with me.

I shall discuss what seemed to contribute to the development and emergence of self in Andrew and what seemed an obstacle. Andrew spent much of the time in his therapy playing out and telling stories and I shall describe some of his changing uses of stories as they reflect his fluctuating developments in self and communication. With one or two exceptions, I have not included theoretical discussion in the clinical description and commentary but have instead given a brief account, near the end, of the psychoanalytic theory on which I have drawn.

Referral

Andrew was referred at the age of 3 years 7 months. At the time of the referral Andrew was in the autistic unit of a special school. The referral came from a consultant child psychiatrist, with a view to assessment for intensive psychotherapy. Andrew had previously been seen for an extended assessment because of language and communication delay and associated behavioural difficulties. These had led to the breakdown of two nursery placements when Andrew was 2 years old.

In the referral, the child psychiatrist wrote that it seemed Andrew's behaviours were somewhat fluctuating and had made professionals think that there might be a strong emotional component to his quite severe communication and interaction difficulties.

The child psychiatrist described Andrew, from his own contact with him, as a restless child who did make some eye contact but who also showed autistic features such as constant twiddling of one object, which Andrew kept spinning round and round, and a sudden 'switching off' of all attention.

Early history

Andrew was born slightly early. His birth was straightforward. For the first seven weeks of life Andrew had extremely bad colic around bedtime, although not at other times, and it had been very difficult for him to get to sleep, although once settled he slept well. From seven weeks he began to sleep very badly and this had continued ever since.

Andrew was breastfed and his mother described him as a guzzler. At three months she introduced some solid food and began to feed him at times with a bottle while continuing also to breastfeed. Andrew had a very strong reaction against feeding from a bottle.

Andrew's parents described his early development as normal except for his speech, which started sometime after the age of one year; out of the blue Andrew had suddenly said a word which wasn't connected with anything that was happening. He developed limited speech, two- or three-word phrases, although there was a feeling that he was capable of more and that his understanding was good. At around 18 months Andrew seemed to stop looking at people and his limited speech development seemed to slow down considerably.

Assessment: initial meeting

A colleague and I met Andrew and his parents for the initial assessment meeting. My first sight of Andrew in the waiting room was of a boy standing on his own, immersed in energetically pushing a toy pram around and banging it quite hard on the floor, in a world of his own. He made no response when we said hello to him.

In this first meeting both Andrew's parents seemed very agitated and quite desperate. Andrew soon picked up a toy car and began pushing it round the room. While my colleague talked with Andrew's parents, I followed Andrew around and commented on what he was doing; I was unable to catch anything from the conversation and I felt as if being together with Andrew cut me off entirely from his parents and my colleague and what they were saying. Andrew spent most of the time on the move, pushing the car round the edge of the room on all the surfaces – wall, table, couch, desk, wall. My colleague was sitting on the couch and I was shocked to see Andrew repeatedly squeeze behind her on the couch and clamber across her back as if she were merely part of the furniture and not a human being, in order to get past and carry on pushing the car in a continuous motion.

Andrew also pushed everything roughly off the edge of the table – cars, figures, toy furniture, plastic containers. He didn't look to see where they landed on the floor. There were two short periods of more concentrated, focused activity. At one point Andrew showed great interest in the doll's house, trying to push a car through the front door and windows and looking inside with what seemed like great curiosity. When I said he seemed to be very interested in what was inside, Andrew immediately said 'Go now' in response, opened the door of the therapy room and started to go out.

Andrew avoided eye contact throughout, apart from two brief moments when he looked into my eyes with what felt like possible curiosity. At one point when he dropped off the front of a chair upside down and head first, I held him as he came down to the floor and Andrew looked at me and smiled faintly.

When I asked anything about what he was doing, Andrew didn't respond. In fact, he barely spoke the whole time except for echoing one or two single words from things I said to him and at the end, when I said 'See you next week', he echoed this with a blank expression in his voice and on his face. When I came out of this meeting my head was literally in a spin.

Assessment: individual sessions

I saw Andrew for five individual assessment sessions. Amidst a great deal of repetitive, cut-off and withdrawn activity, there were occasional moments of spontaneous contact from Andrew. In the waiting room before the first session, Andrew was completely absorbed in 'flying' a toy round and round and up and down; he didn't respond when I said hello but as he came towards me he said 'helicopter'. In the therapy room I said that the helicopter was flying all around and to my very great surprise Andrew replied 'It's looking for somewhere to land'. He spent almost the entire session flying the 'helicopter' round the room, landing it briefly from time to time, then flying it off and round again. He made more eye contact this session and once or twice as he moved about he looked round to see if I was following him.

In the other sessions, Andrew spoke more, often in short sentences that sounded as if they were from stories. He responded to some of my questions about what he was doing and repeated activities from previous sessions each time. He was very preoccupied with what was in the locked cupboards and drawers and repeatedly pulled at them, saying mechanically 'Won't open' and 'What's going on in there?' When I met him for the fourth session, after a two-week gap, Andrew came straight to me and said 'Mr Shulman!' In the last session when he put the telephone to his ear and I commented that the telephone was for people to speak to each other when they're not together, Andrew said 'Hello' into the phone.

Comment

Two features of the assessment seemed prominent. One related to the initial meeting. I was struck by the fact that for the whole hour, Andrew didn't at any time interact at all with either parent. Equally, although Andrew's parents spoke about him, neither parent spoke to him. It was as if Andrew and his parents were in their own, though contiguous, worlds. The second feature was that Andrew was increasingly responsive to the experience of the individual assessment sessions and seemed interested in the kind of contact they offered. It was on the basis of this hopeful sign that three-times-weekly individual psychotherapy was offered.

Fog

In the early months of therapy, particularly at the beginnings of sessions, Andrew usually had a foggy or dreamy air about him. In the waiting room he would be completely immersed in an activity with a toy, often pushing something round on the floor in a world of his own. When I said 'hello' he would straightaway come over to me, as if this were a seamless continuation of what he had been doing and, turning his head and looking away from me, he would mechanically reach out his hand towards mine. At first he didn't actually put his hand in mine, but simply held it out in mid-air so that I could take hold of it. He soon began placing his hand in mine, although it was with no grip and his hand felt weightless and insubstantial. On the way to the therapy room, as he pulled open a swing door (not always the same one) one of his feet would frequently be in the way, stopping him from being able to open the door properly so that he had to move his foot before being able to pass through. He was otherwise well co-ordinated. Andrew would walk along the corridor looking backwards or away from me and run his free hand continuously along the wall and on the banister of the stairs. Sometimes he seemed confused about the way to the room and would turn the wrong way or be about to continue up the next flight of stairs even though he was walking hand-in-hand with me. At other times he clearly remembered the way. At the door of the therapy room he would simultaneously release his hand from mine and open the door with his other hand. Once inside the room he would instantly immerse himself in an activity, usually telling and playing out a story or part of one from the previous session or week.

While telling these stories Andrew seemed to be in a world of his own and one of his own making. He would speak in a storyteller's voice, in single short sentences that he repeated over and over while replaying the same scene. At such times I would usually feel shut out and ignored, with my existence and presence only registered by Andrew insofar as I 'joined' in his story-world by way of asking about details of the story. I would comment about what was happening in the stories and my comments were at times followed either by a development or change of activity, or a move to a new part of the story, although there was no direct acknowledgement of or response to what I had said.

Comment

Andrew appeared at this time to be living predominantly in a world of foggy confusion in which almost everything he did was in the service of creating the illusion of endless continuity; between waiting and meeting, his hand and mine, outside and inside the therapy room, one session or one week and the next, the external world and the world of stories. Andrew's continuous contact with hand, wall and door together with his instant immersion in storytelling, suggest a means of avoiding the frightening experience of separateness and discontinuity. His extreme use of such protective manoeuvres seemed to preclude the possibility of the development of a distinct sense of self.

There was a recurrent state of muddle within Andrew so that, for instance, at times he was confused and could not remember the way to the room. Perhaps in seeking to avoid awareness of being seperate, so that in his mind the distinction between self and other was blurred or lost, Andrew at times lost contact with an important part of himself, namely his memory. Perhaps too there was something in Andrew's mind that actively misled him and sent him the wrong way. There also appeared to be something within Andrew that frequently obstructed his ordinary functioning, co-ordinated self, so that a foot got in the way of the door. Perhaps there was in Andrew's mind the mental equivalent of 'a foot in the way of the door', which led to the physical experience of blocked access.

And then what do you think was happening?

From the beginning I felt that the content of the stories Andrew told had a potential meaning connected with his possible state of mind at the time. For several weeks he was especially preoccupied with a story about a car. Andrew 'narrated' how the car ran out of petrol and came to a stop, the engine wouldn't work and the car was stuck, a kite was attached to the starting handle and flew away with it, chased by the car. Andrew would construct endless different versions of a kite strung to a starting handle, using an infinite variety of toys or bits and pieces from his toy box to represent each, flying them round the room, often spinning himself in a seemingly endless whirl.

When I asked questions about a story, such as who a character was or what happened next, Andrew would now often answer, although if I suggested any possible connection between the story he was telling and himself he would make noises or talk over and drown out what I was saying. For example, in an early session Andrew was playing out a variation on the car story with a boat that ran out petrol and came to a stop. This was followed by Andrew mechanically repeating several times in an exaggerated tone 'And then what do you think was happening?' On this occasion I interpreted this as the car stopping was like his sessions stopping at the end each time and that perhaps he wondered what happened in between. As I said this Andrew made noises that drowned out what I was saying.

Comment

One might think of Andrew's stories as related to experiences of sudden stopping, disconnection, dispersal, loss of control and not knowing, possibly all connected with separateness and separation. However it seemed that even my mentioning him and me not being together, or the gap between sessions, was still intolerable. It was as if there was no differentiation in Andrew's mind between a space for thought about being apart and the space of actual separation. In attempting to obliterate all conscious awareness of separation Andrew obliterated any sense of his own experience of being apart. This had the effect of wiping out the self that had such an experience and the thinking self that might reflect on it.

'We' and 'I'

One marked feature of Andrew's language at the beginning of therapy was his idiosyncratic use of pronouns. At first he frequently used the pronoun 'we' instead of 'I'. He would say 'We need to go to the toilet', 'We need some help', 'We can't do it', 'We want to open it'. Another feature of his use of language was his tendency to give a commentary in brief narrative form, speaking in a storyteller's voice, about what he or I were doing. At first Andrew never, and later only very rarely, spoke in his own ordinary voice. Most of his speech was in the style of a narrator.

Comment

Andrew's use of the pronoun 'we' when referring to himself seemed to be another way of confusing the difference between him as a separate individual on the one hand, and, on the other, him and me as two people together. His narrator's commentary of things he and I did seemed to be an imitative version of my descriptions of what he was doing; but in 'being' or 'being like' someone else, namely a narrator or me, Andrew was unable to be himself. Like Donna Williams in the extract quoted at the beginning of this chapter, Andrew made a story of the external world, as if in his mind he was making things happen by telling them.

Open/hello, close/goodbye

Andrew had, at an early stage, begun a recurrent and more focused activity of opening and closing the room's window. The first time he did this it had followed on from his opening and closing the front door of the doll's house, which I had interpreted in connection with his sessions, coming and going and 'hello' and 'goodbye'. Andrew would close the room window with a bang and I talked to him about how, when we said 'goodbye', he felt he had a bang. In time Andrew began to accompany his opening and closing the window with the words 'Open–hello . . . close–goodbye', which I had originally spoken.

In a session towards the end of the first term of therapy, Andrew at one point opened and closed the window. On this occasion I didn't say anything, waiting to see what would happen. By this time Andrew regularly said the words himself in accompaniment to the action. Andrew said 'Mr Shulman say the words' and I said he wanted me to speak the words for him. The window lever suddenly got stuck and Andrew immediately asked me to help, saying 'Get out Mr Shulman! We need some help . . . We want to close the window'. I said he was saying 'we' but that he, Andrew, wanted me to be a real Mr Shulman who could help him. I suggested that perhaps he might first try to see if he could do it himself. Andrew strained and at first couldn't move it, he became agitated and frustrated but said in a very clear, ordinary four-year-old's voice 'I can't do it'. It was the first time he had spoken in this voice. I talked about what a horrible feeling it was when he wanted to do something but couldn't, and that when this happened he wanted some help. After this Andrew actually managed to free the handle himself and close the window.

In another session around this time, toward the end of the first term, there was some knocking on the wall of the therapy room next door. Andrew looked up alertly and asked in the same ordinary four-year-old's voice 'What's that noise?'

Comment

Andrew now appeared to have 'found his own voice' and to be able to have isolated moments of being himself and speaking as himself. Three factors seemed to make this possible. The first is related to Andrew feeling emotionally more contained and held together: having a therapist think about, understand and put into words his primitive infantile experience of his sessions in terms of beginning and ending, coming and going seems, in turn, to have enabled Andrew to think in a primitive but focused way about an experience of hello/open and goodbye/close. The second factor, in part follow-ing on from the first, is related to Andrew's new occasional tolerance for being aware of a 'not-me' world over which he does not have complete and magical control. Andrew was able to be his ordinary self and to express his ordinary self ('I can't do it'), at the point at which he could acknowledge and tolerate that there was something that, at that moment, he was unable to control. At a deeper, unconscious level I think this related to the idea of a Mr Shulman who doesn't automatically 'say the words', whose speech isn't magically controlled by Andrew opening and closing the window. As a result Andrew had a new sense of a separate 'other' to whom he could express himself. A third factor seems to be the reassurance derived from the fact that there is separate life that is not the product of his own imagination. Andrew could experience and express ordinary curiosity and could speak in his own voice, when there was a noise coming from a child in the next door therapy room.

'Sorry I spoke in words'

In the ensuing months of therapy Andrew would mostly speak to me directly only if he wanted to ask or tell me to do something for him and this recurrently happened in a particular context. He would be immersed and absorbed in a stream of storytelling and accompanying actions, suddenly realise he needed something for his story, come over to me, and deposit on my lap something he wanted tying or sticking, without saying anything. When I did not automatically do what he wanted, he would frustratedly and agitatedly pull at or push my hands as if to make them do it. He was extremely reluctant to use speech to communicate what it was he wanted me to do. While I was doing what he'd asked Andrew would go away from me and spin himself or absorb himself in another activity. When I had finished, he would return to collect whatever it was and immediately go off and immerse himself in playing with it in his story narrative. When this happened I would feel unrecognised as a person, misused if not abused and outraged. I continued trying to encourage him to ask in words and on one occasion when eventually he did so, he violently and furiously thumped the back of a chair to the accompaniment of every syllable he spoke, after which he turned and spoke to a toy animal lying on the floor, saying 'Sorry I spoke in words'.

Comment

Andrew seemed at this time to be intent on avoiding any straightforward expression of need and on actively evading straightforward contact with, and dependence on, a therapist who did things for him. It seemed as if Andrew was a child who psychically had never properly established a dependent infantile self. Instead Andrew appeared to be under the sway of a menacing internal figure whose existence is revealed by Andrew's placatory comment to the toy animal on the floor: 'Sorry I spoke in words'. This frightening and tyrannical internal figure, like a gang-leader, seemed to demand allegiance to a strict code of behaviour: here the non-expression of need or dependence and the non-use of language to communicate, with the threat or eruption of violence in the face of disobedience. This in turn prevented Andrew from relating to me as a person in an ordinary human way.

'The bear wants to stay'

It was following the first holiday break that Andrew began to use stories in a new way. He now started creating and telling his own story vignettes. When I went to the waiting room to collect Andrew for his first session after the holiday he was in a dead sleep and it took his mother and me several minutes to wake him. In the session Andrew played out a brief story that involved a dog that had fallen in the water, went under, and had to be pulled out. Andrew for the first time included me in his play, asking me with a sense of urgency to throw in the life belt and pull out the dog. I was able to talk to Andrew in a way for which he had not previously allowed a space about his wanting me to help pull the dog out of the water and it perhaps being like his wanting me to help bring Andrew out of his sleep and back to life after the holiday.

For some time before the first holiday break I had talked to Andrew about his experience of the ends of sessions and the approaching holiday: his feeling of a 'bang', his not liking to stop or say goodbye, his not knowing what happened in between and his feeling unsure if he would see me again. At the end of this first session after the holiday Andrew placed one of the teddy bears in a cupboard and said 'The bear wants to stay'. Andrew hadn't put away his toy in his toy box and when I asked him to he said clearly and in an ordinary voice 'I don't want to'. It was the beginning of Andrew being able to articulate directly to me, in a variety of ways, his feelings about separation. He started to put toys from the room in his toy box at the ends of sessions and to say 'I don't want to put things away' and 'I want to stay'.

'Larry the lamb wants to go swimming'

A session approaching the second holiday break shows Andrew's developing capacity to use storytelling as a medium for communication. Andrew had missed his last session of the previous week as his class had gone on an outing (I had of course prepared him for this beforehand). Below is a summary of part of the first session the following week.

Andrew started in a very cut-off state. He filled the sink and dropped in the man and woman figures from two toy boats, as well as the fireman from the fire engine, saying they were going for a swim. He fetched the furry lamb and said 'Larry the lamb wants to go swimming. It's Thursday'. He banged the lamb on the cupboard several times, then tried to take it over to the sink to put it in the water. This was something he wasn't allowed to do so I said 'no' to Andrew and he again banged the lamb on the cupboard, this time much harder. For the next few minutes he repeated that Larry the lamb wanted to go swimming and tried various ways to get round me and put the lamb into the water, so that I had to obstruct him to prevent him doing so. I suggested that he was thinking about last Thursday when he didn't come to therapy because he went out with his class. I said he'd wanted to come to his therapy like Larry the lamb wanted to go swimming, that he didn't like it when he couldn't come and felt angry with me, he felt like I had stopped him from having his session just like I was now stopping the lamb from going swimming. Each time I mentioned his wanting to come the previous Thursday Andrew banged the lamb on the cupboard in confirmation.

In a session the following week, approaching the summer holiday break, while I was clearing away at the end, Andrew played out the following scene: he banged two baby dolls with the lamb and said they were crying, and then said 'You can't see Mummy now, you can see her later.' He made the lamb climb on various things in the room. As it climbed over the couch Andrew said 'Bad Mum!' This wasn't something I'd ever said and shortly after – I hadn't spoken in between – he said 'Bad Mr Shulman!' I said he felt I was a bad Mr Shulman therapy mum because he wouldn't be able to see me in the holiday. A bit later Andrew said 'Bad Mr Shulman therapy mum', and after this, 'Mr Shulman built a therapy room'.

Comment

Andrew was beginning to emerge from his isolated and self-isolating world and in his therapy a primitive infantile transference was developing. Tustin (1992) writes of the critical time when an autistic child in psychotherapy 'begins to use situations in the therapeutic setting as equivalents to infantile experiences'. The emotional developments associated with this process seemed to lead to new developments in his communication, play and learning. Andrew's parents reported at this time that they felt Andrew had been with them in a way that he had never previously been and his school reported that Andrew was beginning to learn in new ways.

'I want my mummy'

Andrew had begun to make up quite sophisticated stories and between the summer and Christmas holidays he recurrently told and played out a number of these. Frequently Andrew would repeat and re-tell stories until they were drained of all life and any meaning they originally had. One story involved three animals that lived in a house with a character called Jumping. The animals go to sleep and when they wake up Jumping has gone. The animals wonder where Jumping is, one of the animals 'thought a lot' and the youngest of them says 'I want Jumping', which soon turned into 'I want my mummy'. This latter was always said in an exaggerated mock-whimpering idiot's voice. In a later version the animals had various ideas about what the mother might be doing and what might have happened to her. When the mother returned she would ask what the matter was and what they were so worried about in an exaggerated, uncomprehending voice. I talked about how the animals missed their mummy and wanted to see her again and were worried and frightened when she wasn't there. Also, how it sounded as if there was something wrong with the little one who wanted his mummy so much and how the mummy really didn't seem to understand how worried they'd been.

Comment

In Andrew's internal world the infant that misses and longs for its mother is a subject of cruel mockery; perhaps this is the mockery of an internal cruel gang-leader that despises vulnerability and equates it with handicap and stupidity? At the same time, Andrew seemed to have an internal version of a mother who does not understand her infant's distress about her absence, in stark contrast to his real mother. These features of Andrew's internal world make it much more difficult for him to be able to own and tolerate his vulnerability and his extremely powerful feelings of loss and longing in the face of separation. Instead of being himself Andrew at times becomes an endlessly replaying record and loses himself in relentless perseveration.

'That spells Andrew'

Andrew's placement in a special school had been combined with spending one morning a week in a mainstream nursery. He was approaching his fifth birthday and, as a result of his progress in learning, it was planned for him to start one morning a week at mainstream school. The following is a summary of part of a session shortly after this started.

Andrew took the green felt-tip, wrote on the lid of his paint-box and said 'That spells Andrew'. I said that was his name and that I thought he was showing me what he had learned at school. Andrew looked at me briefly. After this he seemed at a loss to know what to do. He wandered rather aimlessly round the room shaking his hands in the air in a somewhat 'autistic' way. I said it looked like he didn't know what to do after writing his name. Andrew continued walking aimlessly. I said he had left his old nursery and started one morning a week at a new school and that he was learning new things. I was going to continue but before I could say anything further, Andrew went to the sink and very roughly threw all the figures out of the water and onto the floor. I suggested that this was what leaving his nursery had felt like to him – being suddenly and roughly thrown out. [Later] Andrew hid some animals and figures and said 'Where are all the people gone?' I suggested it was like how he might be thinking about the children in his old class at nursery. This led to Andrew playing out a story where a number of animals and figures got into his toy box and had 'a feast'. Andrew said some of the animals 'took the food all the way home'. [Later still] Andrew asked if he could take home a drawing.

Comment

This material suggests a fundamental problem for Andrew about having a sense of himself growing and progressing. Andrew was probably aware of his difference from the other children in mainstream school but I think at a deeper level Andrew had a profound difficulty about the very fact of being there. For Andrew, growth or forward movement seems to be experienced primarily in terms of deprivation. Moving on from the nursery is felt as a violent ejection (the figures thrown out of the water) rather than as progress and growth. At an infantile level Andrew unconsciously seems to equate the children he has left in the nursery with rivals who have stolen the source of nourishment from him (represented in his play by the toy box). These illusory rivals have 'a feast' and take food 'all the way home'. Andrew's unusual wish to take something home thus seems to arise from identification with the stealing rivals. This leaves him without a sense of anything that is really his own.

'Mr I say no'

At the beginnings of sessions Andrew now started running ahead of me to the therapy room so he got in first and, once inside, he banged the door shut on me. At the ends of sessions when I said it was time to clear up he would say 'No!' and 'I don't want to go!' A new story which Andrew played out many times had a 'horrible Mr I say no' character who grunted and went into Andrew's toy box and 'ate all the food' himself. I interpreted that Andrew felt at the ends of sessions or when he wasn't here that I was a horrible 'Mr I say no' who stopped him from being here and who wanted everything here for himself.

There followed a long period during which Andrew was cut off or withdrawn in his sessions, wildly and excitably flying or throwing things round the room, or banging and crashing things down on animals while making noises that were a mixture of panting and gasping, excitement and panic. At times he would immerse himself in poking a hole in a lump of Plasticine and pushing animals through the hole. Often the animals got 'stuck', as had Andrew in endless repetition. He now seemed to have an awareness of what he was doing when he went into these withdrawn states. His parents reported at the time that they also felt this. He also seemed to be doing it more consciously and deliberately. I would often feel quite despairing about whether he was ever going to stop and my heart would sink at the mere sight of him picking up the Plasticine.

I began to talk to Andrew about his wanting to get away from his angry feelings, how I thought he was frightened of them and how he made himself excited to get away from thinking about what he was feeling or what I was saying, and then got stuck doing this. I also started to talk about how when he did this he ended up being on his own and wasn't then able to have the more friendly ' being-together' feeling he had with me at other times. In time Andrew began to respond to these comments of mine, particularly when I drew atten-tion to how he ended up being on his own and he often calmed considerably and was then able to return to what he had been doing before or to start a new activity or piece of play.

Comment

At this time, a year into therapy, Andrew frequently seemed to experience me as yet another particularly nasty and greedy rival for what was his. In such a state of mind Andrew's primary experience of ends of sessions, weekends and holidays was of his access, or even existence, being blocked. Andrew's rage at his growing awareness of separateness and separation frequently took over all else in him and he would retreat into a world of destructive excitement in which he became lost and stuck. However, when I could remind him of the positive experience of being together with me, this increasingly had the effect of bringing him back to himself.

'I'm feeling much better now'

We had to change therapy room after four terms and this provided an opportunity for the further working through of feelings and anxieties linked with moving on. I carefully prepared Andrew for the change and talked about his possible feelings and worries to do with both saying goodbye to the old room and starting in the new one. Following the holiday Andrew slept for the entire first session in the new room but the next session he came with a liveliness I had never seen before. In the waiting room he said spontaneously 'I'm feeling much better now!' and in the therapy room he said 'You can draw a car for me. A yellow BMW. It's got a roof and number plates at the front and back'. This liveliness in the new room ushered in a period of great development and progress for Andrew, characterised by a growing sense of a more sustainable feeling of togetherness. Andrew was now able to remain in contact for much longer periods of time (occasionally whole sessions) and when he did retreat into a withdrawn and cut-off state it was increasingly possible to bring him back.

Much of the time in this period Andrew would ask me in an ordinary way to draw things for him and colour them in and then cut them out. Andrew spontaneously began to join in drawing and also colouring in. This was the beginning of Andrew being able to participate in a consistent way in joint endeavour. At the ends of sessions Andrew began to say what he wanted to do in the next session, and at the start of sessions he would now often ask if he could do something he had been doing the previous one.

Comment

Andrew's developing sense in his sessions of 'going on being' (Tustin 1986 p. 23) seemed partly linked with being helped to think about his experience of a change of therapy room as well as its parallels with the change to one morning a week in mainstream school. Andrew had a new liveliness in the new room. Perhaps my reminding Andrew of both the old and the new room enabled him to have a live sense of looking both back and forward. Andrew thinks of the front and back of a car. Perhaps Andrew has begun at times to feel there is a space in my mind for a memory of him to be kept, like the inside space of a car with a roof. It was at this time that Andrew began drawing three-dimensionally. Andrew also now seemed to be developing a more secure sense of a 'rhythm of safety' that, as Tustin writes, depends on the development of 'an interactive reciprocal relationship . . . with deep infantile roots' (Tustin ibid p.273). This reciprocal relationship in turn stimulated new areas of growth in Andrew.

'And what do you think of that?'

Andrew was beginning to take real pleasure and occasionally even delight both in being together with me and in what he was doing. He now spent much of the time drawing in sessions and gradually did more and more of the drawing himself. He became very interested in tadpoles and the various stages of their growth and he drew many pictures of them. I vividly recall him in one session, drawing a very good tail of a tadpole, something he had frequently found difficult, and saying to me with evident pleasure 'And what do you think of that?'

Becoming a frog

Together with these hopeful developments of self in Andrew there were frequent times when he seemed to 'slip away' or 'slip out of himself'. Often Andrew would start drawing pictures of tadpoles and frogs or chicks and birds. He would then croak and get into a frog posture or make bird noises and flap his arms; he would become more and more immersed in this, increasingly withdrawn and seemingly unable to retrieve himself. I would feel alarmed at the ease with which Andrew could quite literally lose himself. I had previously begun to talk to him about how he seemed sometimes to make himself tired or sleepy to stop himself from having a thought or feeling that was uncomfortable or difficult. Now I spoke about it sometimes being hard for him to carry on being Andrew and to remember he was just pretending or imagining being a frog or bird, that I thought at times he was trying not to be Andrew. When I made these comments Andrew would cry 'Stop that noise, I trying to sleep!' During the fifth term of therapy Andrew elaborated on one particular difficulty in being himself. He had done a series of pictures with a large tadpole and a small one next to it, which we had talked about as a mummy and baby. He then played out and told a story with the cut-out shapes of two large tadpoles and a small one:

> A big tadpole and a baby tadpole were swimming along together. Another big one bumped into the big one with the baby. They all got a fright and turned round and swam away from each other.

After telling the story Andrew became withdrawn and went away to the window, looking anxious. Another recurrent documentary-style narrative which Andrew told and drew pictures for involved large and small fish in the sea, which all ate the same food. The baby fish were always hiding from the bigger ones or swimming away for fear of being eaten by them.

Comment

Andrew appeared unable to experience the ordinary oedipal conflicts because of terrors associated with the early suckling situation in infancy. Tustin (1990) describes this in terms of the infant having an illusory but nevertheless frightening sense of 'danger of being squeezed and jostled out of existence by predatory rivals who are in competition for their "thereness"'. These terrors, she suggests, are subsequently experienced in relation to the father. Andrew's internal version of the oedipal situation seems to be suffused with catastrophe – a mêlée of collision, fear, flight and dispersal. This often led to states of shutdown and withdrawal in sessions and seemed to inhibit Andrew from having a secure sense of self and from being himself.

'I want to be myself'

Towards the end of the fifth term of therapy Andrew told a new story with a depth of feeling and expression that I had never previously heard:

> A chameleon climbed onto different-coloured plants and leaves, each time changing to the colour of whatever he was on. Next the chameleon wanted to be like one animal after another and grew a different part (trunk, long neck . . .) to be like each animal. Then the chameleon was all mixed up. A fly flew past but he couldn't catch it. The chameleon said sadly 'I want to be myself', after which he changed back to how he was originally and was then able to catch the fly to eat it.

When Andrew finished this story I ventured to suggest that he sometimes felt like the chameleon in the story, when he didn't want to be Andrew with all his feelings and that when he tried not to be Andrew he ended up being all mixed up in his mind and wasn't able to think, like the chameleon that couldn't eat. Andrew was far more in contact for the rest of this session and near the end he told another new story, again with real depth of feeling:

> Elsa the elephant was different from all the other elephants because she was 'patchwork'. Elsa says sadly that she doesn't want to be different any more, she wants to be like the other elephants . . .

At the end of the session Andrew sat slumped sadly on his toy box and repeated 'I want to be myself'.

Comment

Andrew is now painfully aware of, and in touch with, his difficulties – in particular the way in which his chameleon self and patchwork self cause confusion and isolation and actually prevent him from being himself. More hopefully perhaps, from the point of view of what might make further development possible, he now has a wish to be 'like the others'. Moreover, Andrew shows an awareness of himself and the ability to express this in a more genuine way through storytelling, which has become creative.

'I need help'

Approaching the end of the second year of therapy, Andrew told a series of stories about babies. Often the baby was in a mess and in one story the baby said 'I can't be seen like this . . . I have to go to talk to Mummy.' Frequently in the stories there would be someone laughing cruelly. Nevertheless, from time to time there appeared an occasional character who was stuck or in a mess and called for help. I picked up on this and talked about the character wanting help and hoping someone would come along. At the end of one session in which Andrew had been particularly reflective, he said in a realistic voice, and with perhaps a trace of resoluteness, 'I've got a lot of work to do'. The following month, approaching the holiday, at the end of a session Andrew said in an ordinary voice 'I need help'.

'You can't catch me'

Andrew's development and progress in learning had reached the point where his placement in special school was no longer appropriate. After a period of planning by his parents and professionals, Andrew transferred to full-time mainstream school with full-time support, following the holiday at the end of the second year of therapy. From several weeks before that holiday and for the next few months after it Andrew repeatedly played out variations of a story involving toy kangaroos. The baby endlessly kept running away from his parents, laughing wildly and saying 'You can't catch me', while the parents chased after him. Andrew would play this out interminably and relentlessly, becoming more and more excited and quite unreachable. I spoke about how the baby seemed to think it was fun running away from his parents and couldn't stop, and that this baby seemed to have forgotten about a nice feeling of being together with his parents. I increasingly intervened to stop Andrew from carrying on doing something that was clearly unhelpful for him. At such times I took away the toys and explained that he could have the animals again when he was able to play properly with them. I also talked to Andrew about how he didn't seem to be able to stop and had got stuck like the baby in the story; that I didn't think it was helpful for him to carry on.

In the waiting room when I went to collect Andrew at the beginning of sessions, he would run away from me and say triumphantly 'You can't get me', or he would try to run round and past me. On the way to the therapy room he began to instruct me bossily to open all the doors. In sessions he would order me to draw the whole of a picture by myself or to put everything away by myself at the end. I had once put into words Andrew's feeling of being left, or told, to do things all on his own (in the context of his first doing new things in sessions and then not wanting to do them) and now Andrew would accompany peremptory instructions to me with the order 'You do it all on your own!'

Comment

Andrew appeared at this time to experience the move to full-time mainstream school not as an achievement of his six-year-old self, but rather as a humiliation of his emerging and developing infant self. He frequently seemed to be completely taken over and dominated by a destructive part of him and appeared to have gone into a manic and triumphant flight from an internal parental couple who are out to get their baby and who are unable to get hold of him. This was then enacted with me in the transference. He feared that I was out to 'get' him and he ran away from me.

In such an internal scenario there is no possibility in Andrew's mind of the parents coming together properly as a nursing couple to look after the infant part of himself. When Andrew was in this state of mind he made it extremely difficult for me to be a helpful or containing figure. Andrew temporarily loses touch with the sane part of himself, which knows he needs help and which would enable him to receive it. He becomes wholly identified with something hostile to his infant self and to his good link with me. In fact, in such a state of mind Andrew does not experience me as a friendly or nurturing figure but rather as a cruel and bullying figure who wants him to do things himself only in order that I can leave him to manage on his own.

'We'll put you outside at night'

Below is an extract from a session approaching half term in the eighth term of therapy. Unusually Andrew's family were going away in the half-term week and he would therefore be missing his therapy. Andrew had been playing out a scene with the toy animals where a baby gorilla hung precariously onto a mother kangaroo's feet in mid-air and kept falling off. I interpreted that perhaps he was feeling the baby part of him wasn't being held properly or kept safe by me here when there was something like a half term. After I said this Andrew began a new piece of play, he tried to put the cup in the doll's house garage but it wouldn't fit. I said there wasn't room for it, it was too big. Andrew then put some of the animals inside the garage and the cup outside, saying in a mocking voice 'We'll put you outside at night. It's best for all the team'. I said a part of him felt I was saying this to him about not coming here in half term, even though the grown-up six-year-old part of him knew he wouldn't be coming because his family was going away. I said he felt I was being a nasty Mr Shulman putting him out at half term, saying he was too big now and there was no room for him and pretending it was good for every-one. Andrew pushed the cup against the open front door of the doll's house, then banged it against the closed door of the garage. I again linked this to his therapy and his feeling shut out and that if he was a grown-up six-year-old Andrew, who could walk and open doors for himself as well as do new, different things, then he felt that the baby part of him was pushed out in a nasty way and that there wouldn't be a place for that part of him too. Andrew's mood changed and he now looked sad. I said I thought he was feeling sad now. Andrew said he would kill his sad feelings and eat them, then went to the couch and turned upside down on it.

Comment

There is a part of Andrew that persistently equates separateness (in the form of greater self-reliance and independence) with abandonment, separation (the half-term break) with cruel exclusion. At home Andrew was regularly going into his parents' bedroom at night and getting into their bed. His parents had to take him back to his own room but Andrew's internal version of this was clearly of a nasty parental couple maintaining a pretence of it being good for everyone, just as his version of not coming to therapy in the half term was of me 'putting him out' for the good of all.

Andrew is unable to have trust in his parents' motives or in mine, which leaves him without the possibility of feeling secure. He seemed to retreat from having a more mature or grown-up self and it became evident over time that he feared something or someone would come along to ruin or spoil anything his grown-up self might achieve.

The king with dirty feet

What followed was a period of several months during which Andrew was preoccupied with things that were damaged and for the first time began to show an impulse to repair or restore things. Andrew now often swung in sessions between a profound sense of despair and inconsolable sadness and a more hopeful sense of putting things right which was accompanied by the growth of a more consistent constructive self. Andrew increasingly turned to narrating stories directly to me without playing them out and the theme of protection emerged. In a session towards the end of the third year of therapy Andrew had been switching off the light, closing the curtains and getting behind them. Following on from this, as well as from a number of other things he had been doing, I had talked to him about trying to protect himself from his difficult or uncomfortable feelings and thoughts by not being Andrew and by shutting things out of mind or putting his mind to sleep. After I said this Andrew told the following story.

> There was a king with dirty feet who didn't like baths and never washed. The smell got so bad that even the king wanted to wash. He went in the river and his assistant Gaboo washed him. The king felt much better but when he stepped out of the river his feet were still dirty. The king gave Gaboo three days to find a solution or he would cut off his head. First Gaboo tried to sweep all the ground but then there was dust everywhere in the air. Next Gaboo tried to wash the ground but then there was water everywhere. Finally Gaboo covered the whole land with a giant carpet so the king was able to walk without getting his feet dirty and was pleased. As the king was walking about there was a man in the crowd who called out 'But if you cover everything then nothing will grow!' The man made the king a pair of shoes. They were the first pair ever made and now everyone wears them.

When Andrew had finished I said I thought this was a very important story and how covering everything up and nothing being able to grow was like shutting everything out of mind and no thoughts being able to grow, that letting some new thoughts grow in his mind could help him to be able to do different, new things and to use his mind to think in new ways.

The fourth year of therapy

I shall give some brief and impressionistic details from the fourth and final year of Andrew's therapy. Andrew was beginning to show signs that he now had a symbolic internal representation of a helpful figure who enabled him to be or know himself. This corresponded with a period when both Andrew's parents and his school reported that Andrew was starting to join in group situations. His parents also reported that at home he had begun playing with his younger brother. During half term of the 10th term of therapy Andrew and his family were away. On his return to therapy he told a story in which an elephant 'lost its head' and was 'in a commotion'. Andrew told a number of versions of this story. Each time he described the head and body of the elephant as having been 'separated'. In each version there was someone who 'will know what to do' and who helped the elephant get his head back on again, after which the elephant said with great relief 'That's better!' I interpreted this in relation to Andrew being away and suggested that it was hard for him to feel he could think properly when he didn't come; perhaps when we were separated he felt a commotion inside like the elephant. Andrew said 'yes!' with recognition. I said I thought he hoped I might be able to help him feel better when he was in a commotion. Andrew again said 'yes'.

Towards the end of the last term of therapy Andrew told an extremely long story which he called 'Spring Clean'. It involved a group of animals in a house:

> At the beginning one of the animals says it's very dark outside. Lion explains that it isn't dark outside but that the windows are very dirty inside. Lion says he is going to do a spring clean and all the other animals moan and complain that it's no fun cleaning. Lion says it can be fun and gets the others to clean while having slides on the furniture and across the floor, which they all enjoy. They clean the mirror and then the windows. At the end they look at the windows and think that they're not clean because it's still very dark. Lion explains that it's not the windows that are dirty but that it's late and dark outside. The animals hadn't realised that they'd been cleaning for so long.

When I commented on the story Andrew seemed to experience this as if I was trying to take away its meaning or value.

Comment

Andrew is able at times now to communicate and express symbolically his inner commotion about a separation as well as his sense of someone who helps him to feel 'in one piece' again. He has the ability to recognise and acknowledge feelings as his own. Finally in 'Spring Clean' Andrew beautifully expresses, symbolically, the story of his own experience of his therapy. This has involved beginning to be able to see and know himself more clearly (the clean mirror) and starting to differentiate between internal and external reality (the dirty insides of the windows and the dark outside). Andrew's sense of self and ability to be himself are still heavily dependent on the presence of an external figure or other (the equivalent of the lion in the story). Andrew is still easily liable to feel threatened by, and in competition with, this other (his apparent experience of me as taking away his own achievement when I comment on the content of his story). Nevertheless his greater capacity at times to be aware of and tolerate separateness has made possible what Frances Tustin refers to as the 'psychological birth' of the child.

Theoretical background

Frances Tustin writes of a 'black hole' type of depression experienced by some infants as a response to what for them was the 'catastrophe of sudden and alarming awareness of separateness from the body of a mother with whom there had been fusion' (Tustin 1992 p.18). She links this with Winnicott's notion of 'psychotic depression' in infants who experience bodily separateness from the mother as a traumatic loss of part of the self (Winnicott 1958). According to Tustin it is this sense in the infant of loss of part of the self that generates the 'black hole' kind of depression encountered in the autistic children she treated by psychoanalytic psychotherapy.

Tustin thus explains psychogenic (in contrast to organic) autism as a protective response to an unbearable and unmanageable psychic catastrophe. Such a response has profound consequences for the development of self in the infant. In particular it precludes the kind of interactive and reciprocal relationship between infant and mother through which a sense of self can develop. Meltzer et al. (1975 p.22) describe this in terms of a 'failure of dependence'.

In *Autistic States in Children* Tustin distinguishes in detail two types of protective response: encapsulation and confusional entanglement. In the first, the autistic child creates a 'shell' or impenetrable 'suit of armour' in order to shut out completely any impingement of the 'not-me' outside world which is experienced as terrifying and hostile. In the second, 'the enveloping and entangling activities of the confusional children . . . draw into themselves the "not-me" in order to confuse and blur it so that it seems less threatening'; here the aim is 'to blunt the child's awareness of needing nurturing care and prevent him from recognising it is separate from himself' (Tustin 1992 [1981] p.128). With confusional entanglement, 'fragments of the self are felt to be dispersed and scattered, so that self and not-self are inextricably confused' (c.f. Andrew's chameleon self).

Tustin picturesquely describes the confusional child as 'a Don Quixote . . . clad in an ill-fitting suit of armour made from miscellaneous bits and pieces insecurely fastened together . . .' (c.f. Andrew's 'patchwork' self (Tustin ibid p.65)). Tustin (1990) describes what she came to understand as the traumatic experience of the early suckling situation for some infants. She suggests that 'these children had a traumatising awareness that the suckling connection was not an ever present part of their mouth'. She continues:

Clinical material indicates that in those moments when the nipple or teat, which was experienced as part of their body, was gone and the babies became aware of their bodily separateness from the suckling mother, they had felt that there were many other sucklings in competition for the object that gave them the mouth sensations which were so vital to their sense of 'being' . . . They feel in danger of being squeezed and jostled out of existence by predatory rivals who are in competition for their 'thereness'. (Tusitn ibid p.48)

In her own discussion (1992 [1981]) of the theoretical aspects of her understanding of autistic children, Tustin discusses the importance of 'primary identification' with the mother or nurturing figure, as a factor in the normal 'genesis of selfhood' and the blocking or confusing of this in autistic children. Here, as elsewhere, Tustin both draws on and refers to the psychoanalytic writing of Esther Bick in relation to infant development (1968, 1986 p.295).

Bick writes about the very earliest and most primitive states of integration and un-integration in the infant. The infant who experiences separateness and separation primarily in terms of catastrophic anxieties, of being 'torn away', 'torn into pieces', 'falling into space' or 'spilling out', may resort to a particular kind of protective strategy which Bick called 'adhesive identification'. This is a primitive form of identification aimed at obviating awareness of separateness, based on the infant having a delusory feeling of being 'at one' with the mother by mentally and/or physically being 'stuck onto' her. Adhesive identification takes the form of 'being-the-same-as' by imitation or mimicry and of 'surface-to-surface' contact, because 'every separation and discontinuity . . . [is experienced as] the unknown third dimension, the fall into space' (Bick 1986).

Tustin suggests that the ordinary development of self can only unfold once these primitive and catastrophic infantile anxieties about separateness have been to a considerable extent contained and worked through. In this way the infant or child comes to have a more secure sense of the parts of the self being held together, in the same way, according to Bick, that the parts of the body are experienced by the infant as being held together by the skin.

Rosenfeld (1987) has written about the way in which the personality can develop a particular 'structure' or 'organisation', which becomes evident during psychoanalytic treatment. The destructive part of the personality can come to dominate and rule over the other parts of the self like the leader of a gang ruling over its members. The 'destructive parts of the self are idealised' and these parts of the self 'are directed against both any positive . . . relationship and any . . .

part of the self which experiences the need for [someone] and the desire to depend on [him/her]'. This prevents the development and growth of the self within the ordinary context of a relationship involving dependency and need, as occurs with infant and mother as part of normal growing up.

Summary

In this chapter I have described the gradual emergence and development of self in Andrew, a four-year-old mild-to-moderately autistic boy, during four years of three-times-weekly psychoanalytic psychotherapy. I have discussed some of the factors that impeded the development of self in Andrew as well as those that enabled him to have a self and to be himself. I have given a brief account of the psychoanalytic theoretical background to my understanding of Andrew, derived from psychoanalytic work with children and adults and from a psychoanalytic understanding of infant development.

Note

The work in this chapter is based on the approach developed by the Tavistock Clinic Autism Workshop.

Chapter 11
Supervision

DIANA SYDER AND CELIA LEVY

Supervision and speech and language therapy – student days and past experiences – the history of supervision in counselling – why is counselling supervision essential? – bringing personal supervision into speech and language therapy – the Sheffield Project – a model of supervision in practice – interpersonal process recall – supervision training – experiences of being supervised.

Supervision and speech and language therapy

There are many different ways of monitoring therapeutic practice and development; they include managerial supervision, personal supervision, appraisal, independent performance review, peer review, case discussions, seminars, conferences, reading, diary keeping, mentoring and discussions. What speech and language therapists tend to understand by the term 'supervision' is 'managerial supervision', or some distant cousin of it, in which sessions are likely to occur infrequently and where the content includes topics such as promotion, career options, time management, goal setting, performance outcomes, and salaries. Such sessions serve as a sort of professional stock-taking and although content and structure may be negotiated between the two participants, they are frequently goal-oriented and judgmental and information may be passed on to higher levels of management.

Personal supervision, on the other hand, which is the main concern of this chapter, is a way of exploring the interpersonal dynamics that operate in any therapy situation. This sort of supervision is not an orthodox part of speech therapy culture. In 1991, Geraldine Rose wrote

256

The question 'What is supervision in speech therapy?' remains unsatisfactorily answered. It is often easier to define what it is not. It is not a system of control where one person has the responsibility of assessing another person's work. It is not merely a support system, nor a form of management or staff appraisal. Perhaps the most important element is the opportunity for regular contact with a person who focuses on you and your job.

In Roberta Green's helpful summary (1992), the aims of non-managerial or personal supervision are stated as being:

- to provide therapists with an opportunity to discuss their work and the demands it places on them;
- to develop an understanding of the interactive processes in relationships with clients;
- to help therapists deal with issues relating to their involvement with clients and with the personal and professional difficulties which can arise from this;
- to protect the interests of clients and ensure that therapists are supported to do this;
- to reinforce and offer feedback on clinical skills;
- to assist the therapist in relating practice to theory and theory to practice and therefore promoting continuing education;
- to offer support to therapists and detect early signs of burnout;
- to challenge therapists on their work practices in a supportive, trusting environment.

In this chapter, whenever the term 'supervision' is used, it is non-managerial or personal supervision that is being referred to. Hawkins and Shohet (1989) explain why clinical disciplines might need to incorporate supervision into their practice:

In choosing to help, where our role is to pay attention to someone else's needs, we are entering into a relationship which is different from the normal and everyday. There are times when it seems barely worthwhile, perhaps because we are battling against the odds, or because the client is ungrateful, or because we feel drained and have seemingly nothing left to give. In times of stress it is sometimes easy to keep one's head down, to 'get on with it' and not take time to reflect. Organisations, teams and individuals can collude with this attitude for a variety of reasons, including external pressures and internal fears of exposing one's own inadequacies.

It could also be argued that not to provide supervision as a regular part of the working week for speech and language therapists exploits this sector of the workforce and may cost dearly in the end.

Self-awareness is a prerequisite for being an effective therapist. It is the gradual and continuous process of developing and exploring aspects of the self: behavioural, psychological and physical, with the intention of developing personal and interpersonal understanding. It is intimately bound up with our relationship with others (Hawkins and Shohet 1993). If we acquire skills without self-awareness we are likely to develop an unnatural and stilted way of operating with our clients and colleagues and we may even feel that our work and non-work selves are poles apart. We are less likely to be able to be flexible with our clients and treat them holistically. Non-managerial supervision is one way of developing self-awareness in clinical settings. It enables us to recognise emotions that are generated in us in response to other people and/or situations and to understand our subsequent reactions. This involves:

- identifying the emotions;
- associating particular feelings with particular aspects of the situation;
- seeing which parts of our own behaviour are generated by which emotions;
- being aware of how our own feelings and behaviour generate feelings and reactions in other people.

'Supervision can be a very important part of taking care of oneself and avoiding feelings of staleness, rigidity and defensiveness which can easily occur in professions where you have to give so much of yourself' (Hawkins and Shohet 1989). It is not the same as team discussion, case conferences or chats over coffee, although all of these do have their own valuable function.

Student days and past experiences

We are most likely to associate supervision with student days, being observed by a therapist and then having to answer her questions afterwards. We may remember being praised for things we did right but we are more likely to remember the therapist's catalogue of our shortcomings being added to our own. That style of supervision brings to mind the way an old friend once described ward rounds when he was a medical student. 'There are two types of ward round,' he said ruefully, 'one where I get jumped on from a great height and another where I get jumped on from a very great height.' It is not surprising that we are often wary of supervision: we may be uncertain of our own abilities and reluctant to put ourselves in a situation where either our peers or our managers are given licence to criticise. We may not wish to re-live the uncertainties of student clinics, or feel we are expected to know more than we do or to have acquired more skills than we know we possess. If we have developed a notion of ourselves as competent therapists, we may see supervision as being likely to challenge that competency or we may be wary of making ourselves vulnerable in a work setting, perhaps because we are unsure of the boundaries between supervision, counselling and teaching. We may feel supervision will wear away at our authority with younger therapists. Some of us may be enjoying our work and may see supervision as unnecessary or only relevant for times when things are not going well or when we have a problem client on our hands – it is easy for our fears of being judged and found wanting to override our desire to develop and learn. We are likely to have pressurised and busy jobs and may regard supervision as one more pressure, or a luxury. We may have been working for a number of years and have developed a style of working with which we are content and find it difficult to see how supervision can have much to offer us. We may simply not know where to go to find it. All the above make us reluctant to embrace the notion of supervision

The history of supervision in counselling

Supervision, as part of counsellor training, has long played an important role in handing on professional skills to future generations. However, supervision of qualified counsellors (practitioner supervision) is a more recent development (Page and Wosket 1994). The British Association for Counselling (BAC) now has made it a requirement of all practising members that they are in supervision, regardless of years of experience. In trying to understand why this is so for counsellors and not for speech and language therapists, the following explanation is posited based on first-hand experience of working in both areas. Speech and language therapists have traditionally been trained in a pedagogic manner, which corresponds to the medical model associated with the practice of the profession. This approach likens students to empty vessels that have to be filled, and when they have been 'filled' they are examined, passed and deemed competent to practise.

In contrast, counselling training has allied itself to an andragogic approach, where students take responsibility for their own learning and aim to become self-directed learners (Knowles 1980).

Counselling tends to be a second career for most people: hence students are usually mature, adult learners and their experience is valued and shared as part of the group learning process. From an andragogic perspective, learning is seen as a lifelong process and, therefore, counsellors are unlikely ever to view themselves as 'finished products': learning from and reflecting on experience are processes that are central to both trainee and practising counsellors' lives. Supervision is the major way in which counsellors in Britain continue their professional development after qualifying (Dryden, in Carroll 1996).

We believe that supervision is as essential to speech and language therapists as to counsellors. An overarching theme in the work of speech and language therapists is loss: loss of the self that might have been; loss of the self that was; loss of function and ability. Although speech and language therapists are trained to be technically skilled to help people recover lost function, the implications of loss and deficit have to be dealt with too. This requires speech and language therapists to make emotional contact with their clients and renders aspects of their work as being not very different from that of counsellors.

Developments in the education of health professionals towards a more student-centred approach and increased awareness of what being a speech and language therapist entails make it the right time to consider implementing a requirement for supervision for speech and language therapists.

Why is counselling supervision essential?

Counselling supervision is:

> A working alliance between a supervisor and a counsellor in which the counsellor can offer an account or recording of her work; reflect on it; receive feedback, and where appropriate, guidance. The object of this alliance is to enable the counsellor to gain in ethical competence, confidence and creativity so as to give her best possible service to her clients. (Inskipp and Proctor 1993, p. 1)

As mentioned above, the BAC insists that counselling supervision is an ethical requirement. 'It is a breach of the ethical requirement for counsellors to practise without regular counselling supervision/consultative support' (BAC Code of Ethics and Practice 1996). Why might this be so?

An important place to begin is to consider what motivates us to be helpers. There is speculation that people are drawn to the helping professions as a way of helping themselves. If this is so and, indeed, there is support for the idea, then most helpers are themselves wounded in some way. Whereas most helping professions encourage helpers to suppress their own 'weaknesses', counsellors are encouraged to be open and acknowledge their wounds. More often than not we can find the motivation behind the need to help in our own stories. Thus lack of care during the childhood of a helper may lead to a compulsive need to care for others. Hawkins and Shohet (1989) believe that it is not the needs themselves but the denial of these needs that can be so costly to counsellors.

So, what needs are fulfilled by being a helper? Hawkins and Shohet (1989) suggest that the answer might include the desire to care, to cure, to heal and the need for power. Supervision provides a context where the needs of the counsellor can be explored so that they are not acted out in the helping process. Secondly, 'counselling is a private and intimate process and experience – for both counsellor and client, in their differing roles' (Inskipp and Proctor 1993, p. 2). As a device, supervision creates the possibility of counsellors being accountable to both the counselling profession and the community at large. It is an effective way of monitoring what goes on behind closed doors. Thirdly, because counselling involves the highly personal world of the client, it may be very demanding on the resources and judgement of the counsellor. The insistence by the BAC that counsellors have ongoing supervision acknowledges the stressful nature of counselling work. Supervision is a helping relationship that exists in part to provide support to supervisees.

Finally, 'the purposes of supervision are the professional development of supervisees and the welfare of clients' (Carroll 1996, p. 8). Thus counselling supervisors have the interests of both the supervisee and her clients at heart. Supervision provides a container within which the relationship between counsellor and client can be supported and maintained. This is not unlike the 'nursing triad' of father supporting mother while she supports her baby (Hawkins and Shohet 1989). The points made above argue that supervision is essential for counsellors. Each argument applies with equal relevance to the speech and language therapy profession.

Bringing personal supervision into speech and language therapy

How might we integrate personal supervision into the speech therapy culture? We can focus efforts on the existing therapists or we can change the expectations of current students so the new culture grows up with them. Concentrating only on the way students operate would seem to be doomed to failure because if the student with her/his fairly fragile values and skills is sent into a culture that does not share those values and the expectations that go with them, then the student/new therapist is likely to adjust her/his thinking to conform with a perceived powerful upper tier. Ideally, we need a two-pronged approach. If students are familiar with exploring their own behaviour and motives in a non-judgmental environment they are more likely to ask for, and gain from, supervision as therapists, and if qualified and experienced therapists and managers are aware of the processes and benefits of supervision they are more likely to attend to their own supervision needs and also to address those of their more recently qualified colleagues. We all need supervision as part of our ongoing development and learning. The way the NHS is structured does not always help us to make adequate provision for the support and learning opportunities we need but it does make it even more imperative that we try to do so. As for the finances, in counselling communities it is normal for counsellors to pay for supervision, in fact some of the psychodynamic training courses make this mandatory, contributing to the high cost of such courses. We could follow suit or provide for it from speech therapy budgets by training speech and language therapists (possibly those who already have a counselling background). We could promote peer supervision, or maybe opt for some hybrid middle ground where therapists pay a percentage and are then subsidised for the remainder by their service. The Riverside Project in the early 1990s, which set up supervision for speech and language therapists, has been well published. Below we describe another experiment in supervision, the Sheffield Project, in which therapists were encouraged to take advantage of local supervision that was both funded and provided by the service.

The Sheffield Project

Organisation

For the years 1992–94, supervision was made available to the speech and language therapy service (60 therapists) in Sheffield. Therapists self-referred and they travelled for supervision to a central location. The supervisor was a speech therapist but had no line-management relationship to any of the therapists except the speech and language therapy manager. All sessions were confidential and if any therapist wished to use material from the sessions with their line manager, that was her/his choice. Supervision was not compulsory but it was free to those who wanted it, funded from within the general service budget. The total number of hour-long sessions was negotiated with the therapist concerned and all therapists were entitled to time-out for supervision.

Issues that brought people into supervision

These fell into three categories: client issues, management issues and personal issues.

Client issues

- I don't know what to do with this client.
- Should I discharge/when to discharge?
- How do I handle situation x?
- Boundaries generally: 'is this part of my job?'
- I want to carry on with this client but I am not sure of my (particularly counselling) skills.
- Why did x happen and what can I do about it?

Management issues

- Balancing demands.
- Personnel management.
- Time management.
- Roles.
- I need to cope with team (intra- and inter-disciplinary) dynamics.
- I'm faced with looking after staff as well as patients.
- I don't get on with my manager/colleagues.

Personal issues

- Too much stress.
- I don't like my job/I want to leave.
- I'm not a good enough speech therapist.
- There are lots of changes going on at work.
- x is happening to me at home and it is affecting my work.

Models of supervision used within the Sheffield Project

As most therapists were unaware of the possibilities, a flexible model evolved that was adjusted depending on the presenting concerns. The initial session was used to get an idea of what these were and to negotiate a style of working:

Model A: Usually a one-off or a short series of sessions using audio/videotaped material though verbally reported material was used where necessary.

Model B: A series of sessions. Often a short series of generic counselling sessions.

Model A was felt to be appropriate for work on specific clients while model B was useful for therapists with stress-related problems or when management issues were a focus. This presented an interesting dilemma. Supervision is not the same as basic personal counselling yet many therapists appeared to request and need just that. It was often necessary to clear away some of the personal undergrowth before the supervision sessions could identify problems and become focused on the original client–therapist relationship. For example, it could not always be taken for granted that when it was necessary to explore issues of control and power between a therapist and client, that the therapist could really understand what was being referred to. It was often necessary to work on the therapist's self-awareness before exploring their thoughts, feelings and behaviours in a specific work situation. For this reason, model B was developed to introduce some generic counselling ideas and as a precursor of client-focused work. Sometimes the two models ran consecutively. There was often a direct and immediate spin-off from personal work into client work. For example, one therapist was feeling useless and hopeless about an elderly, depressed dysarthric client. This was contributing to her own general distressed state. It helped to examine general ideas about loss and what type of support is useful to a grieving person and the therapist was encouraged to generalise from her own experiences to her client. Within a week she reported feeling much more grounded and confident about the support she was giving to the client and consequently no longer avoided arranging to see him.

Benefits of supervision

Feedback was invited from therapists who had taken advantage of supervision. The supervisor had predicted that it would be difficult to assess likely benefits, as with this sort of learning what has been learned may not always be apparent until some time later. However, feedback was surprising in that, as in the example above, it was common to find therapists reporting very rapid changes in how they felt about, and how they were able to work with, a client. This effect has been reported by other supervisors. Here is a selection of general comments about supervision from supervisees:

> . . . a place to 'pull out' and explore my attitudes and emotions about issues and relationships, both with colleagues and patients that are ongoing at work. I have found it incredibly valuable to be able to let off steam with someone who does understand from personal experience but who has no involvement and is not judging me . . . has helped me to see things from other perspectives; sort of taken me out from underneath the problem.

> Having someone to talk through my reasoning behind decisions and check out what personal [biases] have gone into a decision has enabled me to improve the decision.

> Overall I have found that I am being less drained by work now and that means I have more to put back into it.

> Actual sessions need a bit of courage to go through at first. Willingness to make yourself vulnerable. I appreciated the setting down of ground rules especially in relation to employer, confidentiality etc.

> Before supervision I viewed one particular set of clients as 'deadly'. This group was associated with high anxiety for me. After supervision I now view this same group as 'interesting' and don't get anxious about this part of my caseload.

> I benefited from being made aware of my prejudices with a particular client group and working through them.

> I often work with clients who are in devastating circumstances of long-term illness. In order to support them emotionally as well as facilitate communication (the two are inseparable) I need to offload some of the painful issues onto a supervisor who can put things in perspective. The alternative is a dread of such clients or an inappropriate focus on very mechanical, superficial aspects of communication.

> It provided an allocation of time to be objective about my treatment of one of my cases . . . to reflect on our treatment and measure our own standards.

> There was a client who I reacted to with fear and hostility. I didn't feel I could do anything for him. He would not listen to me. Showing a video of a session to a supervisor helped me to identify the client's anger, to accept it and allow it to dissipate by talking it out with the client. If I had not had supervision, I would have discharged him and felt guilty.

Therapists who hadn't taken up the offer of supervision were asked to give written responses for their decision. Here is a summary of comments offered, with the first being by far the most common:

- not enough time;
- other work commitments;
- feeling guilty about taking the time;
- relevant patient no longer attending;
- anxiety that a friendship with the supervisor might interfere with the process;
- put off by the term 'supervision';
- do not need to use it at this stage;
- feeling happy with work life;
- didn't want to end up examining non-work issues in this context;
- pressure;
- difficulty videoing;
- didn't know it was on offer;
- am adequately supported by colleagues.

By the end of the project there appeared to be four clear categories of self-referral:

- therapists considering job changes;
- therapists approximately one-year post qualification. This seems to be a difficult transition time and the most useful intervention at this stage appears to be short-term counselling contracts dealing with generic therapy issues. It is interesting that this is often a time when intense support would be faded out;
- therapists already unhappy in their work who present at times of additional work stress;
- therapists coping with some stress in their personal life that is affecting their confidence and commitment to work.

Stumbling blocks
- It was common to encounter some avoidance when it came to working on individual clients and presenting videotapes. Some therapists were aware of their processes here; others were not.
- There were some misconceptions about the best use of supervision. Word-of-mouth feedback from therapists who did not take up supervision indicated that they felt it was superfluous so long as they were happy and organised in their work. Certainly a prevalent idea is that supervision is for when things

are not going well, for problem clients, or only for times of stress and distress at work.

- Some therapists considered supervision to be a perk and that it should not be provided by the service.

- Some therapists saw supervision as a surreptitious form of counselling and hence not the responsibility of the service. This is an unfortunate misconception, the need to do some groundwork with therapists has already been mentioned and it must be remembered that the wellbeing of both therapist and client is the overall focus in supervision. Any element of personal work with therapists is to this end.

The demand for supervision was equally split between children and adult clinicians with some therapists opting to use video/audiotape, others not.

A model of supervision in practice

Supervision models abound in counselling, where many have their origins in particular theoretical frameworks linked to the practice of counselling – for example, psychodynamic, cognitive-behavioural and humanistic approaches. Currently, literature on supervision in Britain is flourishing. For an up-to-date list of different models of supervision and publications refer to Carroll (1996, p. 11).

In a chapter such as this there is only capacity for a description of one approach to supervision. We have chosen to describe the model proposed by Carroll because it is recent, grounded in practice in this country, and because it addresses the generic tasks of supervision rather than any particular theoretical framework. Carroll's hope is that effective supervisors, regardless of their counselling model, will select tasks appropriate to their supervisee's learning. An outline of the tasks of supervision is followed by an example from practice.

Creating the learning relationship

Supervision comprises a professional relationship, which exists within clearly defined boundaries. There is minimal agreement amongst supervisors as to the exact nature of the relationship: however, all agree that the relationship is determined by the many different roles of supervision. The relationship is also likely to change over time, moving from a beginning phase, which is characterised as a teacher–student relationship, towards a collegiate relationship of greater equality. In order to facilitate learning, creation of safety is an important feature of the supervisory relationship.

Supervision is a working alliance that requires clear contracting and negotiation. Establishing the working alliance is described in detail by Inskipp and Proctor (1993) who stress that both supervisor and supervisee play an equal, if different role, in arriving at the agreement. As the relationship needs to be flexible to meet a variety of needs, each contract is likely to be unique to the particular dyad or group involved. Time and attention need to be given to establishing the relationship and ensuring that it serves the purposes of the supervisee and his or her work context.

The teaching task of supervision

Teaching is an essential component of supervision and enables the supervisee to integrate theory into practice, particularly in the early years after qualifying. Anyone who works within a humanistic framework is likely to view supervision as being about learning more than teaching. Such a model of supervision will be supervisee-centred, and the supervisor's role will be a resource for the supervisee, not an instructor. However, supervision does entail aspects of teaching.

The counselling task of supervision

Counselling and supervision are both helping activities but supervision is different from counselling. When issues arise in supervision that stem from the supervisee's own 'baggage', it may be necessary to explore these, especially if he or she is not currently having counselling. However, the exploration is undertaken only in the interests of the counsellor's professional development. The aim of supervision is to enable the counsellor to do better work, while counselling aims to enable people to live more resourcefully in the wider context of their lives. It is always possible to suggest that a supervisee seeks counselling if the focus of supervision returns over and over again to personal issues.

Monitoring professional/ethical issues as a supervision task

> The professional/ethical task of supervision ensures that clear boundaries are maintained within both counselling and supervision, that both client and supervisee are safe, that accountability is assured and that personal and organisational contexts are given reflective time. (Carroll 1996, p. 64).

This task has been identified as the normative function by Inskipp and Proctor (1993).

What is important to question here is how far the supervisor is responsible for the actions of their supervisees. In Britain, all actors are seen as responsible for their own actions whereas in America, there have been successful suits against supervisors regardless of whether or not they have attempted to stop a counsellor from following a particular course of action.

Monitoring of the ethical standards of practice is an essential ingredient of supervision. Familiarity with the Code of Ethics and Practice of the supervisee's professional association enables monitoring to take place within an appropriate framework.

Perhaps one of the most complex issues for a supervisor is when she suspects that her supervisee is not acting ethically. One solution is to raise the problem in supervision with the supervisee. Another might be for the supervisor to take the issue to her own supervision. The ensuing action might range from a useful discussion of the problem with the supervisee to recommending to the counsellor that she should no longer practise. In such extreme circumstances, if a supervisee ignores the seriousness of the situation, the supervisor may withdraw from the relationship.

The evaluation task of supervision

In certain contexts, supervision may have an evaluative function, for example, in an organisational setting. Where the counsellor is in private practice, periodic reviews may take place whereby feedback is given and received by both supervisor and supervisee.

Complex issues related to power and authority become entangled in a working alliance, which is established to provide safety for the counsellor to explore her work. However, most supervisors feel that evaluation is essential to their practice of supervision and involves challenging work that falls short of good standards. Whether this is tackled formally (in writing) or as an ongoing part of the verbal exchange will depend on the participants and the work context. When the relationship between supervisor and supervisee feels safe and trusting, the supervisee is more likely to bring difficulties or dilemmas to supervision in order to learn from them. Generally, the supervisee is involved in evaluating her own work before receiving feedback from the supervisor.

The consultation task of supervision

This is one of the most interesting and complex tasks of supervision. Consultancy usually refers to the attention given to process in supervision. Hawkins and Shohet (1989) have evolved a 'process model of supervision', which focuses on two interlocking systems: the therapy system and the supervision system.

Focus on the therapy system includes three aspects of the counselling process: reflection on the client's story, the counsellor's interventions and theories, and the relationship that is emerging between client and counsellor. Focus on the supervisory system also includes three areas: reflection on the counsellor's countertransference reactions to the client; reflection on the parallel process of what is going on in the 'here and now' of supervision that may relate to the 'there and then' of the counselling relationship; and reflection on the supervisor's countertransference reactions towards the supervisee and the client.

Most time in supervision is spent on this task. Depending on the developmental stage of the supervisee, time may be spent on different focal points. For example, new or trainee counsellors may benefit from the rigorous discipline of focusing on the first two areas: the client's story and their own interventions. More experienced counsellors may learn more from concentrating on levels three, four and five. Experienced supervisors tend to use level six as a way of tapping into what might be going on in the counselling relationship.

The administrative task of supervision

Counselling always takes place within a context and that context influences the process of counselling. For example, in an organisational setting, factors such as the political climate, differences in values, budgetary matters, and who employs the supervisor will all affect the counselling process. Administrative issues arise even in private practice; for example, taking referrals and dealing with other workers in a client's life. The administrative task involves exploring the implications for counselling of the different contexts in which the supervisee works. In supervision, time may be devoted to enabling the supervisee to deal with difficulties in her work context. When the supervisor is employed by the agency, it is very important to clarify accountability at the outset of the relationship. Will a report to the agency be required? To what extent is supervision confidential? In order to demonstrate how some of the above might translate into practice, in the following section a supervisor illustrates the ways in which the working alliance was established, the administrative tasks tackled and evaluation undertaken:

> When I began working with Jill, a counsellor in a health setting, we spent almost a whole session clarifying how we might work together. What did she want from supervision? First, she wanted to check in and tell me how she was feeling about herself at work. Then we would deal with whatever clients she wanted to present.

She would say at the outset how much time she wanted to spend on each and I would monitor time. She wanted to learn and grow as a counsellor and asked me to be very challenging in my responses to her presentations. She also undertook to tell me if she wanted support at any particular time. Our sessions would last an hour and take place every two weeks. I explained to her that I was in supervision myself and that I presented my supervision practice to my supervisor. This affected the confidentiality that I was offering. We agreed to review our relationship at the end of the first term and conduct a formal, written review at the end of the first year.

Her health centre was paying for supervision. Did they have any expectations of me? How would payment best be effected? In what way was I accountable to the centre? We agreed that I would write a letter to Jill's line manager stating the basis of our contract and requesting agreement before we began working together. I asked that our supervision work would remain completely confidential unless I had serious doubts about Jill's competence to practise. In such circumstances, I would discuss the situation with Jill and then with her manager. I would invoice the centre on a termly basis. If Jill cancelled or failed to attend sessions and I was unable to reschedule them, I would still charge for them. We would meet every two weeks for 40 weeks of the year. I requested that an additional five sessions be made available to deal with any emergencies that might crop up. The manager wrote back agreeing to my terms, but asked that she be notified if Jill did not attend sessions that were charged to them. This was agreeable to me.

At our first review, it became apparent that Jill dreaded being judged by me. It was her first year after qualifying as a counsellor, and she assumed that she should know everything. She had been a nurse before and had this model of training in mind. She felt incompetent as a counsellor and that she was disappointing me.

How important it was to be able to discuss this openly! What emerged from our discussion was an interesting parallel process. While Jill felt inadequate, so did I. This counsellor was receiving great numbers of referrals that were vastly complex, raising challenging ethical dilemmas and involved other health workers in a way that contaminated the counselling relationship. I wondered if my supervision was adequate to support Jill. When we examined what was really in the room between us, we discovered that Jill thought I was all-knowing and confident, while I had an opposite view of myself. I thought Jill was coping brilliantly, while she thought the opposite. We had both been hiding our fears of inadequacy from each other. Both of us had tendencies towards perfectionism and a desire to get things right. Bringing this to light changed our relationship dramatically and we were both able to be more congruent.

Interpersonal process recall

This can be used for supervision and because it is a form that easily lends itself to peer supervision, it has the potential to be useful in speech and language therapy and so is worth describing in some detail. A transcript of a supervision session is given later in the chapter. Interpersonal process recall uses video or audio material. Can you remember the first time someone suggested you make a video of yourself working with a client for the two of you to look at later? The thoughts that leapt into your mind were probably along the lines of 'Oh my God! I can't say no or it'll look as if I'm not keen. I'm supposed to welcome constructive criticism but I hate being criticised! Not only will I have to sit through all the mistakes I already know about but I'll find out about an awful lot more as well. It will be dreadful.' Add to that therapists' horror of having their shortcomings recorded for posterity and a fear of being judged and found wanting by their peers, it is hardly surprising that they rarely leap with enthusiasm at the thought of presenting working tapes or, if they do, they are likely to select segments in which they feel they are presented in a good light. Whatever our initial fears, having feedback through video- or audiotape recordings has been shown to act as a powerful aid to learning (Roe et al. 1978). Familiarity with the experience of seeing oneself on video helps to reduce self-consciousness but we still have to deal with the threat of being judged by colleagues. So how can we get the best out of video and avoid being paralysed by the above? Interpersonal process recall (IPR: not to be confused with independent performance review, a completely unrelated management tool) is a process that uses video or audio material in a nonthreatening way to look at interactions between people. During IPR one can recall throughts, feelings, goals, aspirations, bodily sensations and many other covert processes. It was developed in the sixties by the charismatic American psychologist Norman Kagan and allows people to examine the way they interact with others through the relative safety of a recording. This distancing usually makes it safe to allow learning to occur where otherwise our normal fears might interfere. Clarke (1997) points out the affinity of IPR to person-centred approaches to therapy and education, also that IPR claims to develop 'the internal supervisor'.

A standard IPR procedure would involve making a video of an interaction such as a session between a client and counsellor. After the session – and this can be immediately or days or weeks later – the counsellor replays the tape in the presence of a supervisor who in this role is given the title of 'inquirer'. The supervisee is the 'recaller'. The recaller is given a preamble about how it is not possible to concentrate and process all the things that are happening during a counselling session because there is so much going on, but the video will be a way of slowing things down so that they can be identified and explored. The recaller is asked to stop the tape whenever he or she remembers any thoughts or feelings experienced at that same point in the actual session. The stop button is completely under the control of the recaller. At no point does the inquirer ever stop the tape or indicate that a particular segment would be worth looking at, even if he or she is thinking it! The recaller, on the other hand, stops the tape as often as he or she wishes. Each time the tape is stopped the inquirer helps the recaller's exploration of the event by use of inquirer 'leads'. These are mainly open questions that encourage exploration of issues such as affects, cognitions, body sensations, expectations, mutual perceptions, associations, and unstated agendas. There are four basic sets of responses available to the inquirer (Kagan 1980):

- Exploratory responses: these are open questions and simply help the supervisee recall the issues in the session that were relevant to him/her.
- Checking out understanding: these involve clarification without challenging.
- Focusing on feelings: these responses concentrate on the feelings experienced during the session.
- Honest labelling: these try to get at what was really going on between the participants.

These responses are used to encourage the recaller to reflect on their process of self-exploration, the clients' view of the situation, the therapist's own behaviour, values and assumptions as well as the social and physical environment of the session. Some examples of inquirer leads are:

- What feelings did you have at that point?
- What do you think the client felt when you said that?
- Were you aware of any physical sensations?
- What do you think the client really wanted of you at this point?
- What did you want of the client?
- Can you tell me more about this?
- What effect did that have on you?
- What were you afraid of?
- What did you want the client to say at that point?
- Could you make that clearer for me?

Inquiry requires many skills with which we are already familiar but there are some differences between an inquirer role and a counsellor role. In general an inquirer is less directive, does not use empathic or reflective responses, makes no attempt to interpret and uses a mainly questioning mode of facilitation. Nor are there any direct teaching moments; the inquirer elicits material from the recaller. It can be difficult for trained counsellors to restrict themselves to the inquirer leads as the two sets of skills are close enough to be confusing. It can be very tempting to come out of inquirer mode and become involved in the original issue – in other words, become a counsellor. On work-shops Kagan always stressed that 'It's all too easy to get back to Aunt Matilda rather than staying with the de-briefing and the process occurring between client and counsellor. Having said that, Aunt Matilda, client, counsellor and inquirer are not unconnected.' Kagan insisted that the emphasis must remain on the 'then' of the video session rather than the 'now' of the recall interview. There are some useful variations on the above method:

- *Individual recall.* This is the scenario described above. Of course it is possible for the client to become the recaller with the inquirer. Individual recall has been successfully used in social skills training with brain-damaged people (Heffenstein and Wechsler 1976).
- *Mutual recall.* This is a trio in which both client and counsellor are recalled together by an inquirer. Both counsellor and client can stop the tape. Mutual recall has been applied to other situations such as a teacher, after a class, being recalled together with the class, by an inquirer. It gives insight into the dynamics between the teacher and the class and can be used by teachers wishing to improve their presentation skills.
- *Group recall.* Here a group interaction is taped and the group replays the tape in the presence of an inquirer. Any member of the group can stop the tape at any time. It is a powerful way of quickly getting at the dynamics operating within that group.

Video is the most common medium used in IPR but good work can be done with audiotape. It is not necessary for the inquirer to know the client's background in any detail, or even to be able to see the tape as it is played back and although recallers usually want to put the inquirer in the picture it is advisable to keep this part of the session to a minimum. Kagan warned inquirers against getting too involved in the original material and reminded them instead to remain focused on the recaller's reactions to it.

The basic skills for inquiring can be learned in about three days of intensive work.

IPR yields a huge amount of material for consideration and it is a common finding that 10 minutes of taped material can easily fill an hour's supervision time. In the transcript later in this chapter the supervisor and supervisee watched no more than 10 minutes of tape. The recaller may wish to select segments of the original session to look at but experience suggests that different segments of the original therapy hour will throw up similar issues if an issue is important – if a dynamic is important for the therapist in that session, it will be present throughout the session.

One of the dilemmas for people using IPR is how to deal with material that comes up and cannot be dealt with within the model, say personal issues for the therapist/recaller. It is usually better to keep the boundaries clear and a useful format allows an agreed initial part of a supervision, say 20 minutes, for IPR, after which the participants leave the model and go into another mode of supervision that can deal with the personal issues, or in which overt teaching can be allowed to happen. This is particularly helpful when the recaller is a less experienced therapist with limited knowledge of practical strategies or theory.

Supervision training

Supervision in counselling is becoming a profession in its own right. The BAC Code of Ethics and Practice requires specific training in supervision skills. Supervision training involves:

- Knowledge about supervision, understanding different models, review of ethical and professional issues, and knowing how different professions can interface with supervision.
- Reviewing issues within supervision such as power, gender, cross-cultural counselling and supervision.
- Isolating and practising the skills involved in being a supervisor. These skills would range from setting up supervisory contracts to effective evaluation.
- Understanding and implementing the tasks of supervision. Training here would include the ability to move between different supervisory roles: teacher, counsellor, consultant, evaluator, etc.

- Being supervised for the supervision taking place. This is best carried out in group supervision and allows supervisors to review their own work and learn from their experience and that of others.
- Knowledge of the stages that supervisors go through. Knowledge of such stages can help supervisors monitor their own work. It can also help them anticipate the future and be somewhat prepared for what is to come (Carroll 1996, p. 32–3).

Carroll (1996), among others, stresses that good counsellors do not necessarily make good supervisors. This has important implications for selecting a supervisor and for deciding whether or not to train as a supervisor. Skills for supervision are different from skills for counselling, although there is an overlap between the two. An effective supervisor will be able to structure supervision appropriately, use the counselling role as needed, help supervisees find their own way of being a counsellor, be a good teacher, be flexible, contract clearly, evaluate fairly, adapt to individual differences in supervisees and be aware of cross-cultural issues in supervision, be trained as a supervisor, give feedback clearly and constructively and have access to a variety of supervisory interventions (Carroll 1996, p. 28–9).

Supervision courses vary but when Celia enrolled in 1991 on a training course for counselling supervision run by Cascade practitioners, the course involved attending for four weekend modules spread over six months. Each module had a different focus, and homework was given each time (both written and reading). The aim of the course was to prepare for BAC recognition as a supervisor. It is important to stress that being a supervisor also involves being able to make good use of the supervision process so in the skills practice sessions, feedback was given to both supervisor and supervisee on their use of the allotted time. The course covered all the generic tasks of supervision listed above. More than that, drawing on and sharing experiences with a group of 24 practising counsellors was a wonderful learning experience.

Many establishments that train counsellors now train supervisors too. Courses are advertised in counselling publications such as *Counselling*, which is the BAC journal. One of the 'Catch 22' dilemmas about training as a supervisor is that you need to have current supervisees and to be in ongoing supervision. This might make it difficult for speech and language therapists to join existing courses for counselling supervision and make it more appropriate to establish training courses specifically for speech and language therapists.

Experiences of being supervised

It is easy to talk about supervision – theory, models, practice. As we have already said, many books are devoted to doing just that. It is less easy to give a flavour of what supervision will feel like from the inside; to some extent you have to suck it and see! So we end this chapter with the words of therapists who have done just that, including ourselves. The following accounts are by speech and language therapists who were asked to write about their experience of supervision:

Mary. Supervision has given me a place to 'pull out' and explore my attitudes and emotions about issues and relationships, both with colleagues and patients who are ongoing at work. I have found it incredibly valuable to be able to let off steam with someone who does understand from personal experience but who has no involvement and is not judging me.

Taking the space to look at these situations has helped me to see things from various other perspectives; sort of taken me out from underneath the problem. This has given me the chance to see alternative solutions or at least view the problem from a perspective that makes it seem smaller. I've become less afraid to look into myself and started to know myself better, which has also facilitated the beginnings of self-change. Somehow in this I've started to feel stronger.

It has given me an experience of good, useful counselling, which has certainly started to expand my own range of counselling skills and willingness to take risks in counselling and demonstrated how valuable it really is.

It has also helped with management issues. Having someone to talk through my reasoning behind decisions and check out what personal biases have gone into a decision has enabled me to improve the decision. This has made me more comfortable with it and given me more confidence to present ideas to colleagues. Overall I have found that I am being less 'drained' by work now and that means I have more to put back into it.

Liz. My supervision session provided an allocation of time to be honest about my treatment of one of my cases. Well we do ask about difficult cases or problems with cases and retrospectively to agonise with questions such as: What went wrong? Was that the right thing to do or say? Why didn't I . . .? We generally don't give ourselves time to learn from what we do as standard, to reflect on our treatment or measure our own standards. Supervision appeared to provide time and encourage this self-discipline. I know video would have been helpful if I'd had the time to set it up and the know-how! The logistics were intimidating, let alone then having to watch it with a supervisor!

David. Actual sessions need a bit of courage to go through at first. Willingness to make oneself vulnerable. I appreciated the setting down of ground rules especially in relation to the employer and confidentiality and so forth. I feel I need supervision because of the nature of the relationship I have with clients. For example I can take on a lot of responsibility for a client who is unable to communicate freely. It is difficult then to remain objective about what the client needs from therapy and what it is possible for me to give them. A third party can assist in clarifying not just treatment issues but issues to do with a relationship with the client.

An example was a covert stammerer to whom I reacted with fear and hostility. I didn't feel I could do anything for this client; he would not listen to me. Showing a video of the session to a supervisor helped me to identify the client's anger, to accept it and allow it to dissipate by allowing him to talk it out. If I had not had supervision, I would have discharged him and felt guilty. After identifying the nature of our relationship I had the confidence to negotiate a better outcome with him.

Exploration of feelings with dysfluent clients puts me in a very powerful position over them. I need to be accountable with my feelings and perceptions in order to be aware of dynamics such as transference that could affect the therapeutic relationship. I benefit from being made aware of my prejudices about a certain client group and working through them.

I often work with clients who are in devastating circumstances of long-term illness. In order to be able to support them emotionally as well as facilitate communication (the two functions are hard to separate) I need to offload some of the painful issues onto a supervisor who can put things in perspective. The alternative is a dread of such clients or an inappropriate focus on very mechanical, superficial aspects of communication.

Amanda. When my supervisor first explained the ideas behind her supervision project I thought it sounded like a great idea but somehow it took me a long time to organise my first session. My excuse was being too busy to take time out from clinical work but I was also very apprehensive at the thought of someone probing into my darkest therapy hang-ups. The fact that I am still going after several weeks means that the sessions have felt safe and I've been able to take things at my own pace.

I clearly remember my first session. The setting brought memories of my student days flooding out and after talking things through in the session I realised that I needed to sort out some things from the past before tackling the present. The early sessions concentrated on my experiences as a student, which had continued to affect the way I viewed myself as a therapist. I found these sessions very intense and soon learned not to book in anything else straight afterwards. My colleagues would find me walking around in a world of my own for the rest of the day.

I now see my supervisor every other week as I find this gives more time for the things we have discussed to sink in. I have started taking in tapes/videos of therapy sessions for us to look at together and I still find this quite nerve-wracking as I always have so many criticisms of my own work. Sometimes I go in with a particular client or situation on my mind and am always amazed at the complexities that are lurking behind the 'simple' therapist/client relationship. The insights gained may be very practical (for example, giving the parent a lower, 'comfy' chair may be excluding them from feeling part of the session) or may result in subtle changes in approach (for example getting away from the image of the therapist being in control/responsible for the outcome of each therapy session).

For me, clinical supervision has been a unique opportunity to explore myself as a therapist with someone who knows about the job and is a counsellor. It feels like an immense luxury to take time out and I do sometimes get guilt pangs at leaving my 'real work' to contemplate greater things. Through clinical supervision, however, I hope to become a more effective therapist and if I value my work and myself I will continue to give myself this time. The insights I've gained can be painful and my supervisor is always on hand with the box of tissues, but already I have made inroads in some of the areas I find difficult. It's all about taking risks and so far they have paid off.

Diana. The following is a transcript of an IPR session in which I was being supervised by Peter Clarke who, besides being a long-term friend and colleague, was a clinical psychologist and first introduced me to IPR. We are both watching a tape of a session I had just completed with a man who stammered, although the recall itself could have happened any time over the next few weeks or even months. It was not a counselling session but I had been intrigued by the dynamics operating between this client and myself. In our supervision session I was the recaller and Peter Clarke, as supervisor, was acting as inquirer. Because this tape was intended partly as a demonstration tape, Peter begins by reminding me of the IPR process. As we said earlier, it is not important in IPR for the inquirer to possess the background details of the client and you can see from the transcript that I do not give those details to Peter but, for interest, I had taped myself doing a short session of technique practice with a man who was attending a group run by students. I was supervising the students over a fortnight's intensive clinic. The supervision session helps me to identify what was going on for me and makes me think about what may have been going on for the client, during the original therapy session:

Peter. Just to remind you of the ritual, the point of doing this is to give you an opportunity to think about the original experience with the client on the tape, more fully than you would have time to do at the time, to process and put it into words. When we watch the tape it serves as a prompt to help you bring back to mind stuff you might not be able to bring back to mind. So, things you might not otherwise have had time to say, perhaps risks you anticipated and decided one way or another to act and all sorts of feelings, fantasies and bodily sensations you didn't have words for at the time and perhaps you didn't want to stop to think about. Also queries you had about what was in his mind, things you wanted him to see. All those things. The purpose is to recall and explore what you experienced then and not to attack yourself. So you have control of the recording and if you start playback and whenever you recall anything, whether it seems important or not, relevant or irrelevant, anything that pops into your mind as you watch the tape, stop the tape and we'll explore. OK?

Diana: Yes. Do you want me to set the context or go straight in?

Peter: Go straight in . . . whatever's useful.

Diana: OK. I'll start.

Diana: [Starts and stops tape.] Oh gosh. I have one hundred and one million agendas in my mind here. There's somebody watching through the viewing mirror and this is my 20-minute slot with him and I'm itching to work directly with the client and not have to go via a student. That was a very predictable response he gave. He can be quite difficult, quite hostile and resistant although he controls it as best he can in these situations and I'm thinking 'Oh dear, I want this to be very straightforward.' There are boundaries that I've got in my mind and already he's thrown me a dud card really and I'm trying to make the decision what to do about it.

Peter: Yes. What were the possibilities you were considering at the time?

Diana: He's given me a very uninsightful answer for the level that he's at and I don't know whether to address that and get into the business of setting a hierarchy with him and exploring that or whether to skate across it in order to get on to the material we are aiming to tackle. And another bit of me is thinking 'Uh oh, here he goes again.'

Peter: Mmm. Any bodily sensations? Reactions?

Diana: They were around at the time because I was still anxious because he's just been in a group that's finished and the group over-ran. While I was waiting for them to finish I knew the television wasn't working, so I'd managed to get a technician to come over, but he couldn't get into the room until the group finished so all sorts of things had been going on and I haven't had a few minutes to calm down.[Laughs.]

Peter: Is there anything you did want to say to him at this stage, that you didn't feel appropriate?

Diana: Yes. I think I'd have just liked to say 'Oh, come on! Don't give me that stuff!'

Peter: Yes. Mmm. Do you think he was aware of any of that in you?

Diana: I'm not sure . . . some of his dynamics are complicated and I never personally had the opportunity to explore them, but I think his relationship with me is also complicated. I think he has to prove himself . . . And . . . I'd really like us to get rid of the pressure to do that so we could just do the work.

Peter: Yes.

Diana: And I'm never quite sure how to tackle that one with him. Can we move on, I think that's all?

Peter: Yes. OK.

Diana: [Starts and stops tape.] Oh dear [shaking head]. Nothing is ever where you want it to be. I think I should be able to go in a room, sit in a chair I want to sit in and know things will be to hand, confident that anything I need will be in that treatment room. This is a quick additional session, I haven't had time to prepare the room and there's no picture material in the room and no stopwatch. OK, I should have thought to bring a stopwatch in with me, but I have been doing many other things . . . At this point I'm completely forgetting I've got my own watch on with a second hand! I'm just thinking 'Oh no!'

Peter: What kind of a feeling was that to you?

Diana: Er . . . Really resigned, because the only bits that ever feel safe here are the actual times when I'm in a room with a client and the four walls are the boundaries of what's going on. But on this occasion, even that's not working and I'm thinking 'What's the point? Does it ever work out easy?' It's never easy. That's the feeling somewhere there.

Peter: Somewhere? [Gestures.]

Diana: Yes, here. [Gestures to chest.]

Peter: Here? [Copies my gesture.]

Diana: Yes [Laughs.]

Peter: What's that feeling meaning for you?

Diana: It's frustration and it's 'Oh dear I've got to think of a way out of this . . .'

Peter: Mmm?

Diana: It's irritation because I'm aware we've got a very short space of time here and I'm going to have to go out of the room and think of something.

Peter: Anything you wanted to say to him and didn't?

Diana: Yes. I suppose . . . along the lines of . . . 'I'm really wanting to keep this session very structured' because I think he's more comfortable there and 'I usually try to be better organised than this.'

Peter: Anything get in the way of saying that to him?

Diana: Mmm. Haste. The need to go and do something. Rush.

Peter: I'm wondering what you would have wanted the camera to see or not see at this stage or him to see or not see?

Diana: I would have liked the camera to see a very calm, organised

and structured performance because I was partly wanting to use it as
a model for the student behind the viewing window and maybe for
other students. But instead I'm feeling very hot and thinking about
all the things we've just talked about. I was a bit surprised that I
came in very cool there and got on with it. I suspect I was looking a
bit severe with the effort of controlling it.

Peter: Yes. What did you want him to see at that point?

Diana: Er . . . I think I wanted to set the mood and I wanted him to
see that you do just get on with it, whatever happens . . . He's very
eager and very good at avoiding doing the task and talking a lot
about it instead and I really want to set this model for doing rather
than talking at this point. I'm not wanting to make a big issue about
the watch or tripping over the wire. He's looking at me very quizzi-
cally. I'm not sure about that yet.

Peter: Do you remember what you felt inside when you saw him
looking like that?

Diana: Bit puzzled really because what I'm saying is reiteration, he's
well experienced in this way of working and yet it looks like he's
hanging on my every word . . .

Peter: Yes . . .

Diana: I don't know.

Peter: Was there any awareness in your head about what was going
on in him at that time?

Diana: Er . . . I'm . . . I suppose I was anxious that he would be
getting impatient with the faffing around.

Peter: Mmm . . .

Diana: I think that had been something that had been bothering him
in the previous session with the students and his group and because,
yes, because he's had students working with him and I think he's
quite hard for students to deal with . . . er . . . I don't know, I suppose
a bit of me is wanting to counteract that in some way. Yes, there's a
bit of . . . oh dear, oh dear . . . there's a bit of 'Right. Here we go. This
is the real thing, done properly.'

Peter: OK . . .?

Diana: [Starts and stops tape.] OK, while he's doing the reading, I
think I'm thinking: 'Phew, a breathing space.' I should be concen-

trating on what he's doing. I'm wanting to watch him and listen really carefully but I'm using this space to bring myself down a few levels and tune in to him, so I'm only tuning into him at this point and I should have done that before we started really.

Peter: Mmm.

Diana: There's a slight feeling of relief as well as 'OK, now we can go . . .'

Peter: Is that connected with that feeling here? [Gestures to chest.]

Diana: Yes. Some of the fluttering was starting to go and I was cooling down.

Peter: Mmm . . .

Diana: [Starts and stops tape.] I'm relieved we're actually into it now. Er . . . I'm working really hard here not to rush things. I want to know where his fluency breaks down so I know I want to go up a hierarchy of tasks but I'm not sure if we've got time to do it and I was trying to decide whether to keep him at this rate, 80 syllables/minute or to move him up and do the whole shebang at one hundred.

Peter: Any risks to you in this course of action?

Diana: Yes, if I take him too fast I half predict that his fluency will break down and I sort of think he'll be annoyed with me, because I'm not sure how much he has a need to show me he's OK and can do this stuff.

Peter: Mmm . . .

Diana: The risk of not pushing it is that we don't go far enough and I don't get the information I need out of this session.

Peter: Weighing up those risks, what could that mean for you?

Diana: Er . . . It was crystallising a conflict that had been going on through the whole of this week for me, the whole fortnight . . . Which was about not being free to make my own decisions with the clients about what is going to work for us, because I've had a bevy of students. Four students have been working with this group and the conflict of what the clients need, what he needs, what I need, isn't easy to deal with some of the time and I think I'm wishing 'I wish we'd got an hour. I wish this was my client so we could just mess around for a bit. Wouldn't it be nice.'

Peter: What would you anticipate that would do, if you were able to do that?

Diana: I would have enjoyed it more. Have fewer anxiety symptoms and it would feel more centred around what he needed. Yes, they weren't the only things going on, the other thing is that he's not my client. None of them are. He's in long-term therapy with a colleague and this fortnight has very tight constraints on it. We're here to do technique practice and all the time in the back of my mind . . . oh just get on and get that stuff out of the way. The practice is useful . . . He's in therapy with Eleanor. And I'm feeling that staying within the boundaries of what we've agreed I should do with the students is really frustrating, probably more with him than the other clients I've been supervising. Goodness, there are so many frustrations in my head it's a wonder I'm giving him any attention at all! Mmm . . .

Diana: [Starts and stops tape.] I'm just waiting for him to make a joke, smart crack, a witticism. He loads things. Not only does he expect himself to make a fluent comment, it has to be something smart, so he's not content to be in technique and there's something about his witticisms that . . . It's a bit of . . . and I'm just waiting for him to include the clever comments and at that point his fluency will go.

Peter: Any feelings inside you at this point?

Diana: No. Nothing else at the moment. But I'm sitting back and waiting for it to happen.

Peter: The anticipation is that his fluency will go?

Diana: Mmm. But I remember being surprised when he did go all the way through, it opened up options, but I'm looking very severe. I'm looking very disapproving. I don't think I was disapproving at all . . . I'd actually like to work with this guy a bit more and understand what's going on. I'm still dealing with so many things in my head, trying to understand him and work out what to do with the time that's left. I think it's the concentration that's making me look severe. But I'd rather look encouraging. [Laughs.]

Peter: Any idea what was going on in his mind then? Did he see you as looking severe do you think?

Diana: He's probably expecting – I don't know what he's expecting. The normal routine is to give feedback after fluency tasks, so he'll be expecting that. I suppose he could interpret my dourness as me not being very impressed or pleased with what he's doing, except – I always have the feeling with him that he's actually trying to score in some way. And I think at the moment it's feeling as though he's scored one and that he's pleased about that.

Peter: And how do you feel inside about that?

Diana: Mmm. A little bit of me is pleased he's done it, because it means he's improved over the last few days but, I can't quite articulate it, but I think there's some competing for who is going to be boss.

Peter: Mmm. Is there anything you were wanting to say that didn't seem appropriate? Any fantasies in your head about what you might say?

Diana: Mmm. I maybe would have, in retrospect, liked to say 'I'm very glad you managed to do that.' Also I was busy working out the next task. I wish I hadn't looked so severe.

Peter: At the time, going back to the tape, what were you aware of feeling in your face? Or were you not?

Diana: Still hot. The temperature in the room is hot. I wasn't aware of looking so rigid. I was aware of the time pressure.

Diana: [Starts and stops tape.] Thank God I smiled! A bit of me was thinking then 'If you can predict not having any problems with that one, why on earth, right at the start when I asked you at what point it fell apart, why could you not have given me some indication because you obviously can predict!'

Peter: Is there anything getting in the way of you saying that?

Diana: Yes. He makes me a feel quite irritable and I don't know what that is about and in this rushed setting I'm not sure I could gauge . . . I don't want my irritation to show to him.

Peter: Mmm, what was important to you about not showing that?

Diana: If I show him I'm impatient, no not the same thing, I don't know what his reaction would be and he's quite hostile in many ways. I think there'd be a lot waiting to come back at me and it's outside where I have permission to go. It's a huge area for him is my guess. Vast. I'm obviously picking up the same things other people are but I've agreed not to go in there, these are the boundaries on it and I know we'd be into some fairly major stuff. At the moment it's none of my business.

Peter: So how were you feeling that you weren't able to go there?

Diana: It feels unfinished all the time.

Peter: Mmm . . . [End of segment.]

Peter: Does that feel it's given you something to think about?

Diana: It's reinforced something that has come into my mind on a number of occasions, which is that I should somehow respect the space I need to do certain jobs. Now there are all sorts of very good reasons why it's extremely hard to get that space, but it's the second reminder I've had in a fortnight that the whole thing becomes counter-productive if I don't put some boundaries and find some calm to do that work. Yes, and about the fact that teaching and therapy are different roles that get tangled up in these types of activities.

Peter: In the sense of teaching him? Or teaching the students?

Diana: The students. And I hadn't realised, or I'd forgotten, because I've realised this before . . . you can only hide things so far and when I'm having to make so many decisions in my head and concentrating so hard, I look as if I am. And I always forget how that must come across to someone else, who is probably already uncertain about the way they are going to be received by me! Anything else? Yes. I think it's made me realise how many different things I sometimes try to think about all at once.

Peter: Mmm.

Diana: And that I shouldn't do that to myself or certainly not to the client. That's the main thing. Another layer of reminder that you can only do so many things at once.

Peter: A lot of oughts and shoulds in there . . .

Diana: I know. And at the moment I don't know how to get round the oughts and shoulds because they're very much part and parcel of the way things operate. [Sighs.] That's something . . . there's more than a glimmer of resentment that comes in, that there aren't any answers to some of those oughts and shoulds and I'm put in a position where I have to deal with all this at once.

Celia: While still working as a speech therapist, I began counselling training in 1980, with the intention of extending my skills in working with adults who stammer. During my training, we presented clients on our course, and I began to value other people's input. At work, my two colleagues and I established a peer supervision/support group, which was very important to me. Admittedly, at the time, we were approaching supervision as a means of deciding what to do next with our clients, but the habit of consultation began.

In 1987, I joined a supervision group at the Centre for Personal Construct Psychology. This was very useful in the formative (teaching) aspects but there was little support offered and no input on ethical practice. It did not meet my needs at that time.

Later that year I took the plunge and searched for and found a counselling supervisor who knew little about stammering but practised from a humanistic perspective. I was clear about what I wanted and we made an arrangement that supervision would include training as a person-centred counsellor, plus exploring issues in me that interfered with my work. That year was the steepest learning curve of my counselling career. Suddenly a whole new world opened up. Instead of focusing on the client's issues, I began to tune into what was going on between my client and myself and to understand how this affected our work together. I have continued to have individual supervision since that time, albeit with a different supervisor. In addition, I have formalised a peer supervision arrangement with colleagues at work. As I have moved from speech therapy to counselling as a profession, I have needed more supervision. For me, supervision remains the highlight of my working life. I value the support I receive, the fact that I am always challenged, the space for just me, the sharing and affirmation I receive. I always leave supervision feeling able to get back out there and do my job.

References

Abudarham S (1991) Hypnotherapy in Practice – A Practical Handbook for Health Care Professionals. Birmingham: Association of Hypnotherapists in Health Care.

Als H (1982) The unfolding of behavioural organisation in the face of biological violation. In Tronick EZ (ed.) Social Interchange in Infancy: Affect, Cognition and Communication. Baltimore: University Park Press, pp125–60.

Ausubel DP, Robinson F (1969) School Learning: an Introduction to Educational Psychology. New York: Holt, Rinehart & Winston.

Aronson AE (1990) Clinical Voice Disorders. New York: Brian C Dekker.

Aronson AE, Peterson HW, Litin EM (1966) Psychiatric symptomatology in functional dysphonia and aphonia. Journal of Speech and Hearing Disorders 31: 115–27.

Bachelor A (1988) How clients perceive therapist empathy: a content analysis of 'received' empathy. Psychotherapy 25: 277–40.

Balding J, Regis D, Wise A, Bish D, Muirden J (1996) Bully Off: Young People that Fear Going to School. Exeter: Schools Health Education Unit.

Bamford J, Saunders E (1991) Hearing Impairment, Auditory Perception and Language Disability. London: Whurr.

Bandler R, Grindler J (1979) cited in Gibson HB, Heap M (1991) Hypnosis in Therapy. Hove and London: Lawrence Erlbaum Associates, pp. 70, 99.

Barber TX, Wilson SC (1978) The Barber Suggestibility Scale and the Creative Imagination Scale: experimental and clinical applications. American Journal of Clinical Hypnosis 21: 84–108.

Barkham MJ, Shapiro DA (1986) Counselor verbal response modes and experienced empathy. Journal of Counselling Psychology 33(1): 1–10.

Barsky AJ (1989) Somatoform disorders. In HI Kaplan and BJ Sadock (eds) Comprehensive Textbook of Psychiatry. London: Williams & Wilkins, p2–4.

Barton RT (1960) The whispering syndrome of hysterical dysphonia. Annals of Otology, Rhinology and Laryngology 69: 156–64.

Battle CC, Imber SD, Hoehn-Saric R, Stone AR, Nash ER, Frank JD (1966) Target complaints as a criterion of improvement. American Journal of Psychotherapy 20: 184–92.

Bayne R, Horton I, Merry T, Noyes E (1994) The Counsellor's Handbook. London: Chapman & Hall.

Beck AT, Steer RA, Garbin MG (1987) Psychometric properties of the Beck Depression Inventory: 25 years of evaluation. Clinical Psychology Review 8: 77–100.

Beck AT, Steer RA (1990) Beck Anxiety Inventory. Sidcup: The Psychological Corporation.

Berne E (1964) Games People Play. New York: Grove Press.

Berne E (1967) cited in Heap M (1991) Hypnosis in Therapy. Hove and London: Lawrence Erlbaum Associates.

Berzon B, Pious C, Farson RE (1963) The therapeutic event in group psychotherapy: a study of subjective reports by group members. Journal of Individual Psychology 19: 204–12.

Bick E (1964) Notes on infant observation in psycho-analytic training. International Journal of Psychoanalysis 45: 558–66.

Bick E (1968/1987) The experience of the skin in early object relations. Collected Papers of Martha Harris and Esther Bick. Perthshire: Clunie Press.

Bick E (1986) Further considerations on the function of the skin in early object relations, British Journal of Psychotherapy 2(4): 295.

Bicknell J (1983) The psychopathology of handicap. British Journal of Medical Psychology 56: 167–78.

Binney V, McKnight I, Broughton S (1994) Relationship play therapy for attachment disturbances in four to seven year old children. In Richer J (ed.) The clinical applications of ethology and attachment theory. ACPP Occasional Papers No. 9.

Bion WR (1961) The psycho-analytic study of thinking: a theory of thinking. Paper presented at the 22nd International Psycho-Analytical Congress, Edinburgh.

Blackburn I-M, Twaddle V (1996) Cognitive Therapy in Action: A Practitioner's Casebook. London: Souvenir Press.

Bloch S, Reibtein J, Crouch E, Holroyd P, Themen J (1979) A method for the study of psychotherapeutic factors in psychotherapy. British Journal of Psychiatry 134: 257–63.

Bond T (1993) Counselling, skills and roles. In Bayne R, Nicolson P (eds) Counselling Psychology for Health Professionals. London: Chapman & Hall, pp 8–1.

Boone D (1977) The Voice and Voice Therapy. New York: Prentice Hall.

Bowlby J (1969) Attachment and Loss. Vol. 1: Attachment. London: Hogarth.

Brazelton TB (1992) On Becoming a Family: the growth of attachment before and after birth. (Revised edition.) New York: Delta/Seymour-Lawrence.

Brazelton TB, Cramer BG (1991) The Earliest Relationship: parents, infants and the drama of early attachment. London: Karnac.

British Association for Counselling (1996) Code of Ethics and Practice for Counsellors. Rugby: BAC.

Brodnitz FS (1969) Functional aphonia. Annals of Otolaryngology 78: 1244–53.

Brumfitt S, Sheeran P (in press) The development and validation of VASES: Visual Analog Self Esteem Scale. British Journal of Clinical Psychology.

Buber M (1958) I and Thou (2nd edn.) Edinburgh: T & T Clark.

Bungener J, McCormack B (1994) Psychotherapy and learning disability. In Clarkson P, Pokorny M (eds) The Handbook of Psychotherapy. London: Routledge, pp 365–83.

Burns DD (1980) Feeling Good. New York: Morrow.

Butcher P, Elias A (1983) Cognitive-behavioural therapy with dysphonic patients: An exploratory investigation. The College of Speech Therapists Bulletin, 377: 1–3.

Butcher P, Elias A, Raven R, Yeatman J, Littlejohns D (1987) Psychogenic voice disorders unresponsive to speech therapy: Psychological characteristics and cognitive-behaviour therapy. British Journal of Disorders of Communication 22: 81–92.

Butcher P (1989) Managing Anxiety: A Practical Guide. London: Audio Arts.

Butcher P, Elias A, Raven R (1993) Psychogenic Voice Disorders and Cognitive-Behaviour Therapy. London: Whurr.

Butcher P (1994) Psychogenic voice loss: Psychological features and treatment. Clinical Psychology Forum 69: 2–4.

Butcher P, Elias A (1995) Redefining the Hysterical Conversion Model of Psychogenic

Voice Disorder. Voice and Laryngectomy Special Interest Group Study Day, 2 December. London: St Thomas's Hospital.

Butcher P (1995) Psychological processes in psychogenic voice disorder. European Journal of Disorders of Communication 30: 467–74.

Carding PN, Horsley IA (1992) An evaluation study of voice therapy in non-organic dysphonia. European Journal of Disorders of Communication 27(2): 137–58.

Carroll M (1996) Counselling Supervision: Theory, Skills and Practice. London: Cassell.

Casper J and Colton R (1990) Understanding Voice Problems – a physiological perspective for diagnosis and treatment. Baltimore: Williams & Wilkins.

Childs S (1993) Assertiveness Training for Bullied Students. Unpublished BSc dissertation, University of Sheffield.

Clarke P (1997) Interpersonal Recall in Supervision. In Shipton G (ed.) Supervision of Psychotherapy and Counselling. London: Sage.

Clarkson P (1995) The Therapeutic Relationship. London: Whurr.

Cohn JF, Matias R, Tronick EZ, Connell D, Lyons-Ruth K (1986) Face-to-face interactions of depressed mothers with their infants. In Tronick EZ, Field T (eds) Maternal depression and infant disturbance: new directions for child development. San Francisco: Jossey Bass.

Dalley T (1989) Art Therapy. London: Tavistock/Routledge.

Dalton P, Dunnett G (1992) A Psychology for Living. Chichester: John Wiley & Sons.

Dalton P (1994) Counselling People with Communication Problems. London: Sage.

Davis H, Followfield L (1991) Counselling and Communication in Health Care. Chichester: Wiley.

Ditchfield H (1992) The birth of a child with a mental handicap: coping with loss? In Waitman A, Conboy-Hill S (eds) Psychotherapy and Mental Handicap. London: Sage, pp 9–23.

Dryden W (1992) Integrative and Eclectic Therapy: A Handbook. Buckingham: Open University Press.

Dryden W, Horton I, Mearns D (1995) Issues in Professional Counsellor Training. London: Cassell.

Elbert A, Dinneson DA, Swartzlander P, Chin SB (1990) Generalisation to conversational speech. Journal of Speech and Hearing Disorders 55: 694–9.

Elias A, Raven R, Littlejohns D, Butcher P (1989) Speech therapy for psychogenic voice disorder: A survey of current practice and training. British Journal of Disorders of Communication 24: 61–7.

Elliott R, Hill CE, Stiles WB, Friedlander ML, Mahrer AR, Margison FR (1987) Primary therapist response modes: comparison of six rating systems. Journal of Counselling and Clinical Psychology 55: 223–38.

Ellis A (1977) The basic clinical theory of rational-emotive therapy. In Ellis A, Grieger R (eds) Handbook of Rational-Emotive Therapy. New York: Springer, pp. 14–20.

Erikson M (1923) cited in Waxman D (1989) Hartlands Medical and Dental Hypnosis (3 edn). London: Ballière Tindall, p. 91.

Erikson M (1923) cited in Gibson HB, Heap M (1991) Hypnosis in Therapy. Hove and London: Erlbaum Associates, p. 103.

Ernst S, Goodison L (1988) In Our Own Hands. London: The Women's Press.

Fawcus (1986) cited in Fawcus M (1986) Voice Disorders and their Management. London and Sydney: Croom Helm, p. 25, 37.

Fourcin A, Abberton E (1971) First applications of a new laryngograph. Medical Biological Illustrations 21: 172.

Fraiberg S (1980) Clinical Studies in Infant Mental Health: the first year of life. New York: Basic Books.

Fransella F (1972) Personal Change and Reconstruction. London: Academic Press.

Fransella F, Dalton P (1990) Personal Construct Counselling in Action. London: Sage.

Freud S (1896, 1962) The Aetiology of Hysteria. London: Hogarth.

Gibbons D (1979) cited in Heap M (1991) Hypnosis in Therapy. Hove and London: Lawrence Erlbaum Associates.

Glaser R (1962) Psychology and Institutional Psychology. In Training Research and Education. University of Pittsburgh Press, Science Editions. New York: John Wiley & Sons, pp. 1–21.

Goldberg D (1981) The General Health Questionnaire – 28. Windsor: NFER-Nelson.

Goldberg DP, Williams P (1988) A User's Guide to the General Health Questionnaire. Windsor: NFER-Nelson.

Goldiamond (1965) cited in Dalton P, Hardcastle WJ (1977) Disorders of Fluency. London: Whurr, p. 115.

Goleman D (1995) Emotional Intelligence. London: Bloomsbury.

Green R (1990) Survey of Counselling in Speech Therapy Special Interest Groups. London: Riverside Community Health.

Green R (1992) Supervision Human Communication. Feb, p. 21–22.

Greene M, Mathieson L (1989) The Voice and its Disorders (5th edn). London: Whurr.

Gurland BJ, Yorkston NJ, Stone AR (1972) The Structured and Scaled Interview to assesss Maladjustment (SSIAM) Parts 1 and II. Archives of General Psychiatry 27: 259–67.

Hall DMB (1984) The Child With a Handicap. Oxford: Blackwell.

Harris M (1977) The Tavistock training and philosophy. In Boston M, Daws D (eds) The Child Psychotherapist and Problems of Young People. London: Karnac, 291–314.

Harris T, Lieberman J (1993) The cricothyroid mechanism – its relation to vocal fatigue and vocal dysfunction. Voice Forum: Voice 2: 89–96.

Haselager GJT, Van Lieshout CFM (1992) Social and affective adjustment of self and peer reported victims and bullies. Paper presented at the 5th European Conference on Developmental Psychology, Seville.

Hawkins P, Shohet R (1989/1993) Supervision in the Helping Professions. Milton Keynes: Open University Press.

Hawton K, Salkovskis PM, Kirk J, Clark DM (1989) Cognitive Behaviour Therapy for Psychiatric Problems: A Practical Guide. Oxford: Oxford Medical Publications.

Hayhow R, Levy C (1989) Working with Stuttering. Bicester: Winslow Press.

Heffenstein DA, Wechsler FS. (1981) The use of IPR in the remediation of interpersonal and communication skill deficits in the newly brain injured. Clinical Neuropsychology4(3): 159–143

Hill CE, O'Grady KE (1985) List of therapist interventions illustrated by a case study with therapists of varying theoretical orientations. Journal of Counselling Psychology 32: 3–22.

Hough M (1994) A Practical Approach to Counselling. London: Pitman.

House AO, Andrews HB (1987) The psychiatric and social characteristics of patients with functional dysphonia. Journal of Psychosomatic Research 31(4): 483–90.

House AO and Andrews HB (1988) Life events and difficulties preceding the onset of functional dysphonia. Journal of Psychosomatic Reseach 32(3): 311–19.

Ingham R (1980) Modification of maintenance and generalisation during stuttering therapy. Journal of Speech and Hearing Research 23: 732–45.

Inskipp F, Proctor B (1993) Making the Most of Supervision, Part 1. Twickenham, Middlesex: Cascade Publications.

Jacobs M (1989) Psychodynamic Counselling in Action. London: Sage.

Johnson W, Darley M, Spriestersbach DC (1963) Stutterers' self ratings of reactions to speech situations scale in Diagnostic Methods in Speech Pathology. New York: Harper & Row.

Kagan N (1980) IPR: a method of influencing human interaction. Houston: Mason Media.

Kagan N (1984) IPR: basic methods and recent research. In Larsen D (1984) Teaching Psychological Skills. Brooks Cole: Monterey, California.

Kahn M (1991) Between Therapist and Client: The New Relationship. New York: WH Freeman.

Kelly GA (1955) The Psychology of Personal Constructs. New York: WW Norton & Co.

Kelly GA (1995) The Psychology of Personal Constructs (reprint). London: Routledge.

Knowles M (1980) The Modern Practice of Adult Education: From Pedagogy to Andragogy. New York, Cambridge: The Adult Education Publisher

Lankton C (1980) cited in Gibson HB, Heap M (1991) Hypnosis in Therapy. Hove and London: Erlbaum Associates.

Lave J (1988) Cognition in Practice. Cambridge: Cambridge University Press.

Laver JD (1980). The Phonetic Description of Voice Quality. Cambridge: Cambridge University Press.

Liss-Levinson WS (1982) Clinical observations on the emotional responses of males to cancer. Psychotherapy Theory, Research and Practice 19(3): 325–30.

Margolin C, Byrne B, Holst-Goltra P (1992) Hypnosis for Pain Control Workshop. 12th International Congress of Hypnosis, Jerusalem.

McFadyen A (1994) Special Care Babies and their Developing Relationships. London: Routledge.

McLeod J (1994) Doing Counselling Research. London: Sage Publications.

Mearns D, Thorne B (1988) Person-Centred Counselling in Action. London: Sage.

Meltzer D, Hoxter S, Weddell D, Wittenberg I (1975) Explorations in Autism. Strathtay Perthshire: Tavistock/Routledge.

Miller L, Rustin M, Shuttleworth J (1989) Closely Observed Infants. Trowbridge: Redwood.

Mitchell L (1987) Simple Relaxation. London: Murray.

Morley M (1969) Disorders of articulation: theory and therapy. British Journal of Communication Disorders 4(2): 151–65.

Mowrer DE, Wahl P, Doolan SJ (1978) The effect of lisping on audience evaluation of male speakers. Journal of Speech and Hearing Disorders 43: 140–8.

Nabuzoka D, Smith PK (1993) Sociometric status and social behaviour of children with and without learning difficulties. Journal of Clinical Psychology and Psychiatry 34: 1435–48.

Neary A, Joseph S (1994) Peer victimisation and its relationship to self concept and depression among schoolgirls. Personality and Individual Differences 16(1): 183–6.

Nelson Jones R (1989) The Theory and Practice of Counselling Psychology. London: Cassell.

Nelson-Jones R (1993) Practical Counselling Skills (2nd edn). London: Cassell.

Nichols KA (1993) Psychological Care in Physical Illness. London: Chapman Hall.

Norcross JC, Arkowitz H (1992) The evolution and current status of psychotherapy integration. In Dryden W (ed.) Integrative and Eclectic Therapy: A Handbook. Buckingham: Open University Press, pp 1–40.

Olweus D (1980) Familial and temperamental determinants of aggressive behaviour in adolescent boys. Developmental Psychology 16: 644–60.

Page S, Wosket V (1994) Supervising the Counsellor: a Cyclical Model. London: Routledge.

Parkinson K, Rae JP (1996) The understanding and use of counselling by speech and language therapists at different levels of experience. European Journal of Disorders of Communication 31: 140–52.

Pervin K, Turner A (1994) An investigation into staff and pupils' knowledge, attitudes and beliefs about bullying in an inner city school. Pastoral Care in Education 12(3): 16–21.

Prater R, Swift R (1990) Manual of voice therapy. Texas: Pro Ed.

Prevezer W (1991) Musical interaction. Speech and Language Disorders 37: 10–11.

Raphael-Leff J (1993) Pregnancy: the inside story. London: Sheldon.

Rathus S (1973) A 30-item schedule for assessing assertive behaviour. Behaviour Therapy 4: 398–406.

Ravenette AT (1977) Personal construct theory: an approach to the psychological investigation of children and young people. In Bannister D (ed.) New Perspectives in Personal Construct Theory. London: Academic Press, pp 252–80.

Ravenette AT (1980) The exploration of consciousness: personal construct intervention with children. In Landfield AW, Leitner L (eds) Personal Construct Psychology: Psychotherapy and Personality. New York: John Wiley, pp 36–51.

Reid K (1989) Bullying and persistent school absenteeism. In Tattum D, Lane D (eds) Bullying in Schools. Stoke-on-Trent: Trentham Books.

Rigby K, Slee P (1991) Bullying among Australian school children: reported behaviour and attitudes towards victims. Journal of Social Psychology 131: 615–27.

Rigby K, Slee P (1993) Dimensions of interpersonal relating among Australian school children and their implications for psychological wellbeing. Journal of Social Psychology 133(1): 33–42.

Robertson SJ (1982) The Robertson Dysarthria Profile. Bristol: Communication Skills Builders Inc.

Roe P, Goldberg D, Jones S, Hyde C, O'Dowd T (1978) The value of feedback in teaching interviewing skills to medical students. Psychological Medicine 8: 695–704.

Rogers C (1951) Client-Centred Therapy. Boston: Houghton-Mifflin.

Rogers C (1967) On Becoming a Person. London: Constable.

Rogers C (1980) A Way of Being. Boston: Houghton-Miffin.

Rose G (1991) Supervision. RCSLT Bulletin June, pp. 5–6.

Rosenberg M (1965) Society and the Adolescent Self Image. Princeton: Princeton University Press.

Rosenfeld H (1987) Impasse and Interpretation. London: Tavistock/Routledge. p. 106

Rowe D (1983) Depression: The Way out of Your Prison. London: Routledge & Kegan Paul.

Scott J, Williams JMG, Beck AT (1989) Cognitive Therapy in Clinical Practice: An Illustrative Casebook. London: Routledge.

Shapiro MB (1961) A method of measuring psychological changes specific to the individual psychiatric patient. British Journal of Medical Psychology 34: 151–5.

Sharkey EA, Manning WH (1987) The effects of emotional arousal and increased speaking rate on children's newly learned /r/ productions. British Journal of Communication Disorders 20: 51–60.

Sharp S, Smith PK (eds) (1994) How to Tackle Bullying in Your School: a practical handbook for teachers. London: Routledge.

Sharp S (1995) How much does bullying hurt? The effects of bullying on the health, happiness and educational progress of secondary aged students. Educational and Child Psychology 12(2): 81–8.

Sheehan JG (1975) Conflict theory and avoidance-reduction therapy. In Eisenson J (ed.) Stuttering: A Second Symposium. New York: Harper & Row, pp 97–198.

Silverman E (1976) Listener's impressions of speakers with lateral lisps. Journal of Speech and Hearing Disorders 41: 547–52.

Simonton C, Matthews-Simonton S, Creighton J (1978) Getting Well Again. Los Angeles: JPTarcher Inc.

Sinason V (1992) Mental Handicap and the Human Condition: new approaches from the Tavistock. London: Free Association.

Sinason V (1993a) The vulnerability of the handicapped child and adult: with special reference to mental handicap (learning disability). In Hobbs CJ, Wynne JM (eds) Child Abuse. Baillière's Clinical Paediatrics, Vol. 1. London: Baillière Tindall, pp 69–86.

Sinason V (1993b) Understanding Your Handicapped Child. London: Rosendale.

Skord KG, Schumacher D (1982) Masculinity as a handicapping condition. Rehabilitation Literature 43(9–10):s 248–89.

Smith PK and Sharp S (eds) (1994) School Bullying: insights and perspectives. London: Routledge.

Snaith RP, Constantopoulos AA, Jardine MY, McGuffin P (1978) A clinical scale for the self-assessment of irritability. British Journal of Psychiatry 132: 164–71.

Spiegel H (1976) cited in Rowley DT (1988) Hypnosis and Hypnotherapy. London: Croom Helm, p. 66.

Spitzer RL, Endicott J, Fleiss JL, Cohen J (1970) The Psychiatric Status Schedule: a technique for evaluating psychopathology and impairment in functioning. Archives in General Psychiatry 23: 41–55.

Stern D (1985) The Interpersonal World of the Infant. New York: Basic Books.

Stern R, Drummond L (1991) The Practice of Behavioural and Cognitive Psychotherapy. Cambridge: Cambridge University Press.

Stokes J (1987) Insights from psychotherapy. Paper presented at the International Symposium on Mental Handicap, Royal Society of Medicine, 25 February 1987.

Thompson CK, Shapiro, LP, Roberts MM (1995) Treatment of sentence production deficits in aphasia: a linguistic specific approach to /wh/ interrogatives, training and generalisation. Aphasiology 7: 111–33.

Thompson DA (1995) Two years on: problems in monitoring anti-bullying policies in schools and their effect on the incidence of bullying. Paper presented at ECER conference, 14–15 September 1995, University of Bath, UK.

Tonge D (1992) Assessing the effects of assertiveness training on victims of bullying in three Sheffield schools. Unpublished BA dissertation, University of Sheffield.

Tustin F (1986) Autistic Barriers in Neurotic Patients. London: Karnac.

Tustin F (1992) Autistic States in Children (revised edition). London: Tavistock/ Routledge.

Tustin F (1990) The Protective Shell in Children and Adults. London: Karnac.

Van Riper C (1973) The Treatment of Stuttering. Englewood Cliffs, New Jersey: Prentice Hall.

Wambaugh JL, Thompson CK (1989) Training and generalisation of agrammatic aphasic adults' WH interrogative productions. Journal of Speech and Hearing Disorders 54: 509–25.

Watanabe H (1994) The application of attachment and amae to clinical problems in Japan. In Richer J (ed.) The clinical applications of ethology and attachment theory. ACPP Occasional Papers No. 9, pp 36–43.

Watkins (1971) cited in Heap M (1991) Hypnosis in Therapy. Hove and London: Lawrence Erlbaum Associates, p. 84.

Watzlawick P, Weakland J, Fisch R (1974) Change: principles of problem formation and problem resolution. Norton, New York. Cited in Hayhow R, Levy C (1989) Working with Stuttering. Bicester: Winslow Press, p. 6.

Waxman D (1989) Hartlands Medical and Dental Hypnosis, London: Ballière Tindall (3rd edn).

Webster WG, Poulos MG (1989) Transfer Strategies for Adult Treatment Programs. Tuscan, Arizona, USA, Communication Skill Builders.

Wellington J (1993) The Work Related Curriculum. In Funnell P, Muller D (eds) New Developments in Vocational Education. London: Kogan Page, Ch. 4.

White A, Dreary IJ, Wilson JA (1997) Psychiatric disturbance and personality traits in dysphonic patients. European Journal of Disorders of Communication 32: 307–14.

Whitney I, Smith PK (1993) A survey of the nature and extent of bully/victim problems in junior/middle and secondary schools. Educational Research 35: 3–25.

Whitney I, Smith PK, Thompson DA (1994) Bullying and children with special educational needs. In Smith PK, Sharp S (eds) School Bullying: Insights and Perspectives. London: Routledge, pp 213–43.

Williams D (1992) Nobody Nowhere. London: Corgi.

Wilson PH, Spence SH, Kavanagh DJ (1989) Cognitive Behavioural Interviewing for Adult Disorders. London: Routledge.

Winnicott DW (1958) Collected Papers: through Paediatrics to Psychoanalysis. London: Tavistock.

Wolpe J (1973) The Practice of Behaviour Therapy. Oxford: Pergamon Press.

Worden JW (1991) Grief Counselling and Grief Therapy (2nd edn). London: Routledge.

Yalom ID (1980) Existential Psychotherapy. New York: Basic Books.

Yalom ID (1989) Love's Executioner and Other Tales of Psychotherapy. Harmondsworth: Penguin.

Index